AGE
Joyfully

How to live
your best life

Publications International, Ltd.

Fitness consultant and model: Katie Morgan

Photographer: Christopher Hiltz

Interior and cover art: Shutterstock.com

Louis Weber, CEO
Publications International, Ltd.
8140 Lehigh Avenue
Morton Grove, IL 60053

ISBN: 978-1-64558-121-5

Manufactured in China.

8 7 6 5 4 3 2 1

This publication is only intended to provide general information. The information is specifically not intended to be substitute for medical diagnosis or treatment by your physician or other healthcare professional. You should always consult your own physician or other healthcare professionals about any medical questions, diagnosis, or treatment. (Products vary among manufacturers. Please check labels carefully to confirm that the products you use are appropriate for your condition.)

The information obtained by you from this publication should not be relied upon for any personal, nutritional, or medical decision. You should consult an appropriate professional for specific advice tailored to your specific situation. PIL makes no representation or warranties, express or implied, with respect to your use of this information.

In no event shall PIL or its affiliates or advertisers be liable for any direct, indirect, punitive, incidental, special, or consequential damages, or any damages whatsoever including, without limitation, damages for personal injury, death, damage to property or loss of profits, arising out of or in any way connected with the use of any of the above-referenced information or otherwise arising out of use of this publication.

CONTENTS

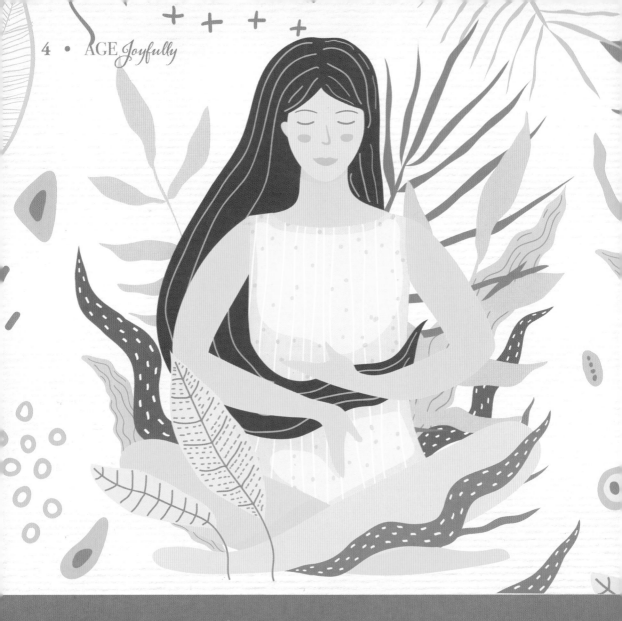

INTRODUCTION

Every eight seconds or so, someone in the United States celebrates their 50th birthday. Blowing out so many candles doesn't seem like such a phenomenal feat today, but it certainly was a century ago, when it was common to die well before age 50. Infectious diseases, such as typhoid fever and influenza, took a heavy toll in those days. Thanks to modern science and technology, we are living longer and longer. What a difference the twentieth century has made!

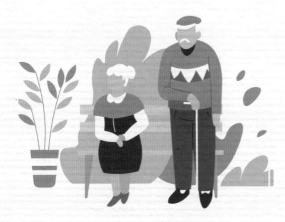

Of course, increased longevity doesn't come without a downside. As you age, you become increasingly susceptible to chronic illness, including heart disease, osteoporosis, cancer, and arthritis. Medical breakthroughs and life-prolonging tactics can help you live a better life that's as free from disease as possible. But medicine can't do it alone. A healthy lifestyle is your greatest asset. Health habits are formidable weapons against the effects of time. What you eat and drink, whether you drink alcohol or smoke, and how physically active you are all greatly influence your risk of disease. In their 40s, 50s, and 60s, people often began to reevaluate their lifestyle in order to prepare for the decades ahead. Fortunately, it's never too late to reach for better health.

Enter *Age Joyfully*, a guide to slowing down and reversing the more unpleasant effects of aging, so that you can focus on the benefits of aging and enjoy retirement. *Age Joyfully* explains what to expect from your body as you age and what steps you can take for peak performance and energy so that you can continue to be active and vibrant. You'll learn what nutrients you'll need more of as you age, how exercise can protect not only your body but your brain, tips for keeping your memory sharp, and more.

Let's face it: Bodies don't get better with age. And while no amount of clean living can guarantee a longer, happier life, chances are your quality of life will be enhanced by better nutrition, exercise, and activity. Pianist and composer Eubie Blake once said, "If I knew I was gonna live this long, I'd have taken better care of myself." *Age Joyfully* will help you live without that regret.

Age Joyfully is not meant to replace the expert advice of your doctor or other licensed health care professional. It is meant as a guide to better maintaining your health for the rest of your life, and it's designed to help you cope with the body changes brought on by the passage of time. Its advice will help you live a longer, healthier, more fulfilling life.

WHAT YOU NEED TO KNOW ABOUT AGING

There are few physical differences among a group of first graders. But if you check out the same group 65 years later, their physical differences will likely outnumber their similarities. Some will be the epitome of health, while others will be managing one or more chronic conditions. Some will be vigorous, while others will be lethargic.

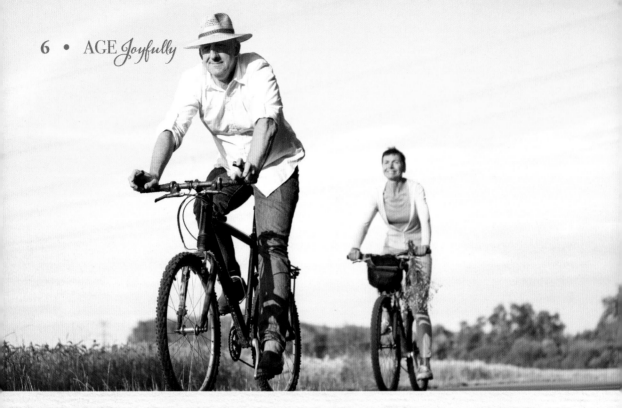

As we get older, we become physically less like our peers. That's because we are the sum of our life experiences. At age six, not too much has happened to our bodies to make us radically different from our peers. But by middle and old age, we've had decades to develop and maintain habits that have an impact on our health, both negatively and positively. The environment, too, affects our health, including where we work and live and how much exposure we have to infectious diseases. Aging is universal, but each of us experiences it in different ways.

HOW OLD IS OLD?

Aging may be inevitable, but the rate of aging is not. Why and how our bodies age is still largely a mystery, although we are learning more and more each year. Scientists do maintain,

however, that chronological age has little bearing on biological age. The number of candles on your birthday cake merely serves as a marker of time; it says little about your health.

NATURE OR NURTURE?

The complexities of getting older make it difficult to pinpoint why one person ages well while another looks and acts older than his years. Are good health and fortitude passed down like green eyes or brown hair? Or are they a product of the environment, including the food you eat, whether you have been exposed to harmful chemicals or infectious diseases, and how much you exercise? Both certainly play a role, but we don't yet know which has a more powerful influence.

Genes are powerful predictors of health and longevity as well as disease and death, but they're only part of the story. If your parents and grandparents lived well into their nineties, chances are you will, too—but not if you abuse your body along the way. (Scientists say all genetic bets are off once you've made it to age 80, however. After that, family history has little bearing on longevity.) And if your father died young of a heart attack or your mother had breast cancer, you may be genetically predisposed to those diseases. Scientists are continually discovering more genetic determinants of chronic and fatal diseases.

While genes partially determine who will develop chronic conditions that hasten the aging process, such as cancer and heart disease, there is no question that a healthy lifestyle is your weapon against the genes you've been dealt, or your ace in the hole if you've got good genes. A man whose father and brothers died from heart disease in their forties and fifties may very well escape the same fate by exercising regularly and keeping his blood cholesterol levels and body weight in check.

On the other hand, a man with no genetic predisposition to heart disease can certainly create heart problems by eating a high fat, artery-clogging diet and leading an entirely sedentary lifestyle.

Healthy living delays many of the body changes that aging brings. And it's never too late to start on the road to better health.

Eating a nutritious diet goes a long way toward insuring good health. For instance, getting enough calcium and vitamin D at any age will retard the onset, and the progression, of osteoporosis, a bone disease that causes pain, fractures, hospitalization, and even death in the elderly. If you're a smoker and you quit at any time, you decrease the chances of having a heart attack. And exercising or becoming more physically active improves lung function and lowers the risk for heart attack, no matter how old you are.

HOW DO WE AGE?

Cells, the most basic body unit, are at the center of any discussion about aging. You have trillions of cells, and they're organized into different tissues that make up organs, such as your brain, heart, and skin.

Some cells, such as those that line the gastrointestinal tract, reproduce continuously; others, such as the cells on the inside of arteries, lie dormant but are capable of replicating in response to injury. Still others, including cells of the heart, nerves, and muscles, cannot reproduce. Some of these non-reproducing cells have short life spans and must be continually replaced by other cells in the body. (Red and white blood cells are examples.) Others, such as heart and nerve cells, live for years or even decades.

Over time, cell death outpaces cell production, leaving us with fewer cells. As a result, we are less capable of repairing wear and tear on the body, and our immune system is compromised. We become more susceptible to infections and less proficient at seeking out and destroying mutant cells that could cause cancerous tumors. In fact, many older adults succumb to conditions they could have resisted in their youth.

Though cell death is the basis for understanding the aging process, it is not the only factor. The aging process is incredibly complicated, and it's often difficult to distinguish between changes that are the result of time marching on and those that come with common medical conditions, including high blood pressure and heart disease. Aging is the inevitable decline in the body's resiliency, which ultimately leads to dwindling powers, both mental and physical. Some aging changes affect us all. For example, diminished eyesight that necessitates reading glasses is considered normal, primarily because it affects everyone who lives long enough. On the other hand, cataracts, which are formations on the lens of the eye that cloud your vision, can be prevented and are not considered part of the aging process, despite their prevalence in older people. To further complicate matters, organs age at different speeds. That's why a 50-year-old may hear as well as someone twenty years his junior, but may have arthritis or high blood pressure.

Theories abound about the underlying cause of aging. Some maintain that aging is preprogrammed into our cells, while others contend that aging is primarily the result of environmental damage to our cells. In this book, we'll focus not on the causes but on common effects and health risks of aging. We may not know exactly why aging happens, but fortunately we have some good ideas about how to age healthily.

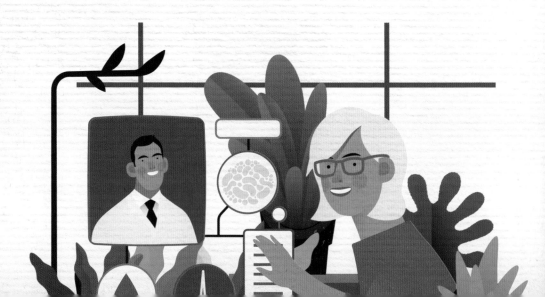

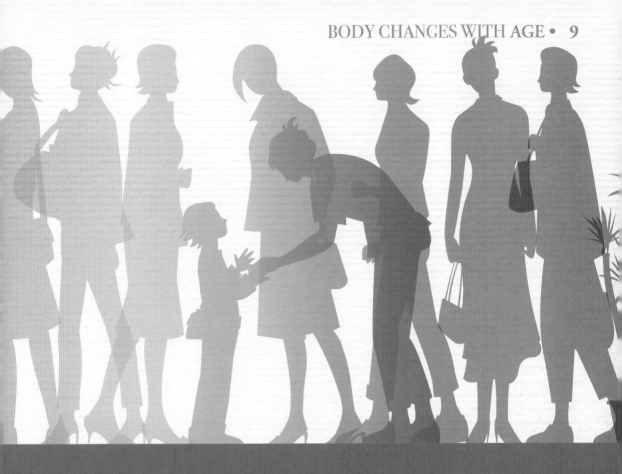

BODY CHANGES
WITH AGE

Some age-related physical changes are obvious: an extra laugh line or two, graying hair, and additional weight around the midsection, for instance. But many changes, such as the gradual loss of bone tissue and the reduced resiliency of blood vessels, go unnoticed, even for decades. Even though you're not aware of them, they're happening, nevertheless.

Knowing how and why your body changes with age will help you discourage alterations in cell, tissue, and organ function that slow you down. This knowledge will also help you take steps to stop the development of conditions such as diabetes and eye disease that are more common with advancing age.

Since it's beyond the scope of this book to describe every alteration aging has in store, we've decided to concentrate on the major body changes that you may be able to delay—or even prevent—by living a healthy lifestyle.

BONE LOSS

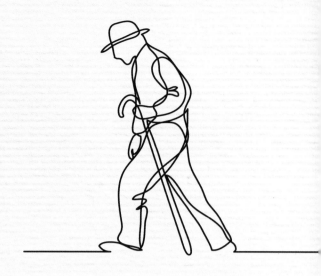

Bones are deceptive: From the outside, they appear hard and stagnant. But bones are bustling with activity. Their tough exterior conceals a vast network of blood vessels that transport nutrients to, and wastes away from, working bone cells. Bones are constantly being remodeled; they are in a continuous cycle of destruction and renewal until the day you die.

The problem is, as time passes you lose more bone than you make. As a result, bones thin and become increasingly susceptible to fracture. As this process accelerates after age 50, osteoporosis becomes more common. Osteoporosis is a condition of progressive bone loss that is painful, disfiguring, and debilitating. It weakens bones to the point that fracture comes easily. Even coughing, tugging on a cabinet door, and especially falling, can cause a fracture in those who suffer from advanced osteoporosis.

Some bone loss with age is unavoidable, but the rate at which bone is lost is highly individual. Genetics plays a role in the development of osteoporosis—Caucasian and Asian women are more likely to develop osteoporosis, as are those who have relatives with the disease. Menopause is also a culprit: Bone loss accelerates in the five years or so after menopause. Bad habits, such as smoking and excessive use of alcohol, also contribute to bone loss, as does a sedentary lifestyle and inadequate intake of calcium and vitamin D. Certain medications such as cortisonelike drugs and cholestyramine, a drug to lower blood cholesterol levels, also accelerate bone loss. So do some medical conditions such as rheumatoid arthritis. However, much research proves that regularly performing weight-bearing exercise, such as walking and lifting weights, and getting an adequate amount of calcium and vitamin D can keep bones strong longer, building bone and reducing the risk of osteoporosis, even in the elderly.

If you think you're shrinking, you're probably not imagining it. We're tallest by the end of our forties, then lose up to two inches in height by age 80. The loss in height is gradual but accelerates late in life.

Why do we get shorter with age? There are myriad reasons including weaker muscles; water loss; postural changes; and deterioration of the spongy disks separating the vertebrae in our backbone, causing a compression of the spine. Women tend to lose more height than men because they are more often the victims of osteoporosis, which results in loss of bone tissue in the vertebrae of the backbone, compressing it and making you shorter. That's why it's so important to maintain bone health and strength throughout life. And it doesn't hurt to sit up straight, either.

JOINTS, CARTILAGE, AND MUSCLES

Joints become less resistant to wear and tear with time. That's in part because of the changes in cartilage, the tissue that cushions the tips of the bones in your joints. Aging causes cartilage to lose water, making it more vulnerable to injury from repetitive motion and stress. Arthritis is characterized by pain and stiffness in the joints, and in some forms, swelling, redness, and heat. It is more common with each passing decade. Osteoarthritis, the most common form of arthritis, occurs when cartilage begins to fray and decay. Osteoarthritis is usually confined to hips, knees, spine, and hands.

Carrying around excessive weight aggravates osteoarthritis in the knees and hips, which bear weight. In fact, being overweight increases your risk of developing osteoarthritis. Regular physical activity may help reduce joint pain and stiffness and increase flexibility, muscle strength, and endurance.

You may have noticed that you can't lift heavy loads nearly as well as you could five or ten years ago. That's because aging causes a decrease in the strength, size, and endurance of muscle tissue, perhaps due in part to decreased blood flow to muscle tissue. But don't put less strength and tone down to age: Inactivity wreaks much more havoc on muscles than time does. Sitting around accelerates muscle loss. In fact, experts say the loss in strength and stamina that we take for granted with old age is in part caused by reduced physical activity. By age 75, one in three men and half of all women get no regular exercise, which exacerbates the muscle loss that age causes.

CALLING ALL COUCH POTATOES

Up until a few decades ago, researchers thought that loss of muscle strength with age was as sure as death and taxes. But more recent research shows how wrong that assumption was. Even nursing home residents in their eighties and nineties can get fit, so you can, too. Ten seniors in a nursing home in suburban Boston lifted weights three times weekly for about two months. In that short time, the participants became stronger, started walking faster, and improved their balance. Two even threw out their canes. And they boosted their bone mass and built muscle, too.

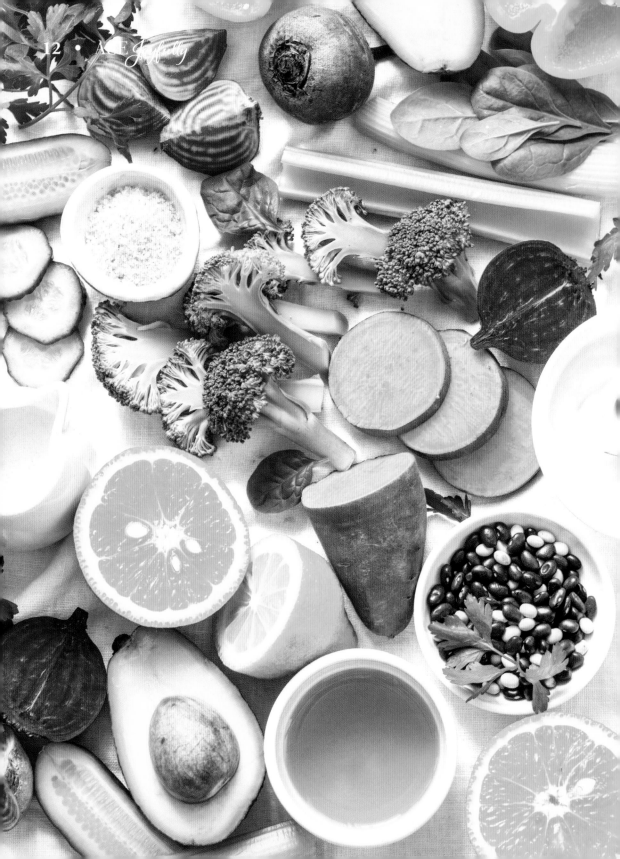

SKIN

Skin is composed of two main layers: the epidermis, the layer you wash and dry, and the dermis, which lies directly below its more visible counterpart and is where hair and sweat glands originate. Dermal and epidermal cells diminish in aging. The dermis actually thins by about 20 percent, and the blood supply to it drops off with time. Wrinkles develop, primarily due to a loss of collagen, a cementlike protein that holds cells together. When it goes, so goes elasticity, the property that provides skin with its resilience, helping you avoid laugh lines and crow's feet in your youth. Sun exposure, too, is a major contributor to the development of wrinkles. In fact, the sun causes most skin damage, including brown "age spots" and skin cancers.

As skin gets thinner and less elastic, it becomes more fragile, bruising and tearing more easily and taking longer to heal. The loss of some sweat and oil glands from the dermis may result in chronically dry skin. Thinning skin also compromises its ability to act as a barrier to infection. Skin injuries, more common with age, also increase your vulnerability to infection.

Aesthetics aside, thinning skin has implications for your health. Your skin participates in the body's vitamin D production. Vitamin D is calcium's partner in helping keep bones strong. It gets its start in skin that's been exposed to strong ultraviolet light. Since aging skin has a limited capacity to initiate vitamin D production, vitamin D deficiency is more common in older people, especially those living in northern climates, where the sun is too weak to make vitamin D for half the year. Applying a sunscreen with a Sun Protection Factor (SPF) of 8 or higher helps protect your skin but blocks much-needed ultraviolet rays.

CARDIOVASCULAR CHANGES

Aging brings on increased stiffness of the chest wall, diminished blood flow through the lungs, and a reduction in the strength of your heartbeat. (In fact, maximum heart rate per minute declines with each year and can be estimated by subtracting your age from 220.) Don't worry too much about this, though. Your heart pumps more blood per beat to compensate for a diminishing heart rate.

Older people take longer to recover from stress, a shock, or surprise. After exertion, such as exercise, more time passes before your body returns to its resting heart rate and blood pressure. Older people often feel colder than their younger counterparts, largely due to diminished circulation.

Blood vessels change, too. Artery walls slowly thicken and become less elastic, increasing their vulnerability to normal wear and tear. While arterial thickening is considered normal, it may predispose you to the buildup of plaque inside your arteries. Plaque restricts the flow of blood to the heart and the brain, which can lead to heart attack or stroke.

Plaque buildup increases with age but is exacerbated by elevated total cholesterol levels and by elevated LDL (low density lipoproteins, the "bad" cholesterol) levels in the blood. A diet rich in saturated fat and cholesterol and low in fiber coupled with a sedentary lifestyle contribute to high blood levels of total cholesterol and LDL cholesterol.

Until about age 50, men have higher blood cholesterol concentrations than women. That's thought to be the result of the protective function of estrogen, a female hormone that helps keep blood cholesterol levels in check. Even when estrogen levels fall and blood cholesterol levels rise after menopause, women still run a lower risk of heart attack and stroke from clogged arteries than their male peers. Because they haven't been suffering from the same damaging high cholesterol levels as men, women suffer from heart attack and stroke an average of ten years later in life than men. But once menopause starts, a woman's risk for

heart attack and stroke rises steadily with each passing year.

Between 40 and 50 percent of people over the age of 65 have high blood pressure, yet scientists are not sure why. In about 95 percent of the cases the cause remains a mystery. The decreased elasticity of the blood vessels as we age may be at least partially responsible for high blood pressure, but lifestyle may be equally, if not more, responsible. Studies show that less technologically advanced countries have virtually no high blood pressure with advancing age, while industrialized nations such as the United States show a steady increase in blood pressure.

Why does it matter? Elevated blood pressure harms blood vessels. You may feel fine, but out-of-control blood pressure is an insidious condition that puts you at greater risk for stroke, heart disease, kidney failure, and other ailments.

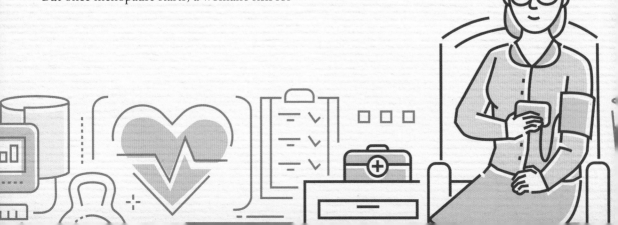

GASTROINTESTINAL CHANGES

You may not think of your mouth as being part of the gastrointestinal system, but in fact, it's the very starting point of the process by which you digest foods and absorb nutrients. As you age, chewing can become more difficult. You may chew more slowly, and you may not chew your food as efficiently. That's especially true if you have dentures or poor dentition. Chewing is important, though, because it breaks down food so that stomach acid and intestinal enzymes can better attack it, digesting it to its smallest components to be absorbed by the intestine. When you swallow larger pieces of food, it takes about 50 to 100 percent longer for it to make its way to your stomach because your esophagus, the pipe that connects your mouth with your stomach, doesn't contract as forcefully as it did when you were younger. As a result, you are also more vulnerable to choking. Slowing down and chewing food thoroughly will help you make the most out of your eating experience and help eliminate some of the problems caused by gulping larger chunks of food.

As many as 30 percent of Americans over the age of 60 do not produce enough stomach acid because of two conditions: hypotrophic gastritis (reduced production of stomach acid) or atrophic gastritis (the absence of stomach acid). You may not feel either of these conditions, but their effects are real. Too little stomach acid results in faulty vitamin B12 absorption. A deficiency of vitamin B12 in your bloodstream and tissues can lead to pernicious anemia and irreversible nervous-system impairment and may contribute to high levels of homocysteine in your blood. High homocysteine is one of the risk factors for heart disease.

People over age 60 have a greater risk of developing gallstones, perhaps because of the narrowing of the bile duct at the opening of the intestine. A high fat diet also puts you at

ACCENTING ACUITY

Want to retain all your faculties later in life? Control your blood pressure now. That's the conclusion of a study that pinpoints mid-life high blood pressure as the major reason for thinning nerve tissue and reduced brain volume of people in their seventies. Researchers found that along with cigarette smoking, excessive alcohol consumption, and poorly controlled diabetes, high blood pressure speeds up the normal changes seen in the aging brain. The take-home message? Get your blood pressure checked regularly. And if it's high, do all you can to get it under control.

greater risk. When you digest fat you need bile, a substance made by the liver and stored in the gallbladder. Gallstones form when liquid stored in the gallbladder hardens into rock-hard material.

Can't stomach dairy? It could be your age. As you get older, you produce less lactase, the digestive enzyme that breaks down the carbohydrate in dairy products known as lactose. It's difficult to pinpoint how many older people can't tolerate the likes of milk, cheese, and ice cream. But if you have bloating and discomfort beginning within hours of eating dairy products, you probably have some diminished tolerance for lactose.

Lactose intolerance is individual. That's why you may be able to tolerate some dairy products and not others. For example, many people with lactose intolerance can eat yogurt, which is lower in lactose than a glass of milk. In addition, consuming milk or other dairy products with food helps to decrease the effects of lactose intolerance, as does consuming smaller amounts at a time.

As you get older, your gut—particularly your colon—may become sluggish and less toned. One in three people age 60 or older have diverticula, which are outpouchings in the lining of the large intestine. These pouches are the result of increased pressure within the intestine caused by decreased muscle tone. In addition, when your gut gets sluggish, you become more vulnerable to constipation.

TAKING HEARTBURN TO HEART

Heartburn is a misnomer: It's got no more to do with your heart than it does with your foot. But it has plenty to do with getting older.

Occasional heartburn may be due to overeating or consuming an irritating substance, including chocolate, peppermint, fatty foods, coffee, alcoholic beverages, citrus fruits, or pepper. But chronic heartburn is probably due to a condition known as gastroesophageal reflux disease, or GERD, which results in the return of the stomach's acidic contents back into the esophagus (reflux).

Reflux occurs when the muscle connecting the esophagus and the stomach weakens, which can happen with age. As if the pain and irritation weren't enough, chronic heartburn can cause esophageal cancer. People who have heartburn, reflux, or both at least once a week are at risk for esophageal cancer; those suffering from the same symptoms at night have an even greater chance of developing the disease. If you're having frequent or chronic heartburn that you can't quell with medication, or if you're having trouble swallowing, talk to your doctor.

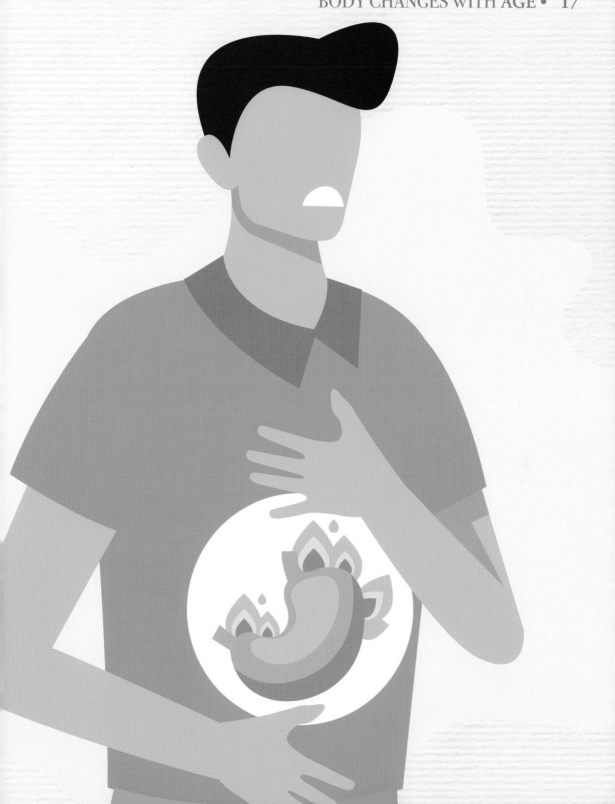

YOUR LIVER

Your liver is your largest internal organ, weighing in at about three pounds. But it gets smaller with time, beginning around age 50. The liver's shrinkage begins at the same time that body weight and muscle mass start their decline. However, in the very old, the liver becomes disproportionately small. Having less liver tissue and decreased blood flow to this organ means that your body may handle certain medications differently. That's why the older you get, the more often you and your doctor should evaluate the effect of all of the medications you take and discuss your alcohol intake.

You can't live without it, but you probably know little about why your liver is so important. The liver:

- makes bile, which helps you digest fat

- helps determine the amount of nutrients that are sent to the rest of your body

- stores glycogen, a complex carbohydrate that is converted to sugar and released into the bloodstream, providing fuel for your body when your blood sugar level falls

- synthesizes many proteins

- processes drugs that have been absorbed by the digestive tract into easy-to-use forms for the body

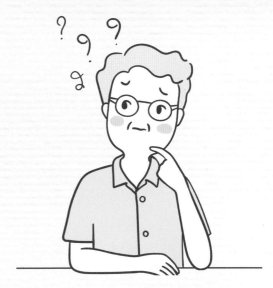

- detoxifies and gets rid of substances that would otherwise be poisonous, such as the waste products from the breakdown of medications and alcohol

ULCERS

With time, you may become infected with Helicobacter pylori (*H. pylori*), a pesky bacteria that hitches a ride on the stomach lining and is the cause of nearly all ulcers. Ulcers are sores or holes in the lining of the stomach or duodenum, a part of the small intestine. They cause pain when the stomach is empty, such as between meals and in the wee hours of the morning, but irritation can come at any time. Sometimes the pain lasts for minutes; other times it hangs around for hours. Eating or taking antacids may relieve your distress, but only temporarily.

H. Pylori infects about 60 percent of American adults by age 60, but infection with the bacterium does not necessarily mean you will develop an ulcer. However, the presence of *H. Pylori* does increase your chances because it weakens the protective mucous coating in the digestive tract and makes it vulnerable to the corrosive effects of stomach acid. *H. pylori* infection is easily cured with antibiotics, sometimes in combination with acid-suppressing medication to alleviate the symptoms and heal the ulcer.

How will you know if *H. pylori* is plaguing you? Your health care provider can use any of the following tests to diagnose *H. pylori* infection:

* **Blood tests:** A blood test can confirm *H. pylori* infection.

* **Breath tests:** This involves drinking a harmless liquid and having a sample of your breath tested one hour later to detect the presence of *H. pylori*.

* **Endoscopy:** A small tube with a camera inside is inserted through your mouth and into the stomach to look for ulcers. During this procedure, small samples of the stomach lining can be gathered for testing for *H. pylori*.

KIDNEYS

You've got two of them, and boy, are they a busy pair. All the blood in your body is constantly filtered by the kidneys, which determine the elements to keep and those to eliminate in urine. Without adequate kidney function, you would not be able to clear toxic byproducts of normal metabolism or those of medication breakdown. Nor would you be able to regulate water balance and blood pressure. Functioning kidneys actually participate in bone health, too, by finishing off vitamin D production that begins in the skin and by regulating calcium and phosphorus loss in urine.

When you're born, each kidney tips the scale at a shade more than 1.5 ounces. As you grow, so do they—to about nine ounces a piece. But as you age, they begin to decrease in size. By your eighties, they've shrunk to about six ounces each. Kidneys also gradually become less efficient at filtering your blood and making urine, beginning around age 30. And as you get on, less blood makes it to the kidneys.

While scientists agree that kidney function drops off with age, they can't agree on why. It could be that you lose nephrons, or kidney cells, and this decreases the organs' capabilities. Some say that undetected infection, injury, and medication reactions and a decrease in blood flow caused by vascular disease may be the reason that kidney function flounders. Whatever the cause, you can preserve kidney function by drinking plenty of fluids; controlling cardiovascular disease, including high blood pressure, as much as possible; and keeping blood glucose levels in check, especially if you have been diagnosed with diabetes. Chronically high blood glucose destroys the tiny blood vessels that supply the kidneys, causing cell damage and death.

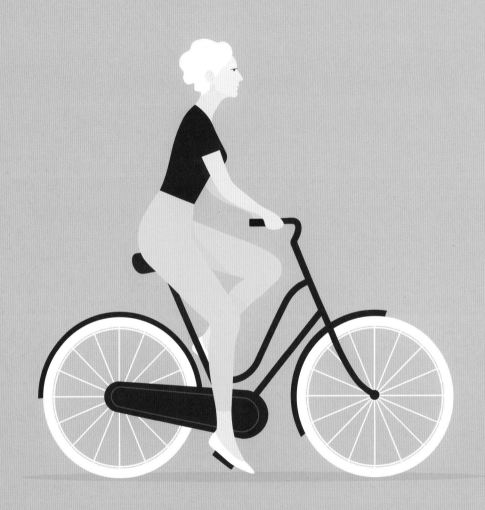

IMMUNITY

The immune system is nothing short of a massive army at the ready, defending the body 24 hours a day. A sophisticated network of cells and organs stationed around the body protects you from invaders such as bacteria, viruses, fungi, and parasites. This network produces and houses the materials to fend off any threat to good health, including the cell production gone haywire that can evolve into a cancerous tumor. What the immune system can't repel, it seeks out and destroys.

If the immune system is an army, white blood cells are the enlisted soldiers. White blood cells and the antibodies they produce are the workhorses of the immune system. They make their rounds via your bloodstream. When invaders enter the body, or when mutant cells are formed, your body mounts its defense by generating a specific antibody. Antibodies are produced by white cells residing in your spleen and in your lymph nodes. An antibody can finish off germs or bad cells, or it can earmark them for destruction by a type of white cells called macrophages, which are responsible for engulfing and destroying unwanted cells.

Aging decreases immunity by impairing the body's production of antibodies. Fewer antibodies means a more sluggish immune system that's less responsive to foreign elements and to potential cancer cells.

There's a little-talked-about organ that scientists say may be the key to preserving immune function. It's the thymus gland, and unfortunately, it takes a hit with advancing age. When you're born, the thymus gland weighs up to about half a pound, but it shrinks to a fraction of an ounce by age 60. In short, it virtually disappears. But we may need the thymus gland to help prevent our immune system from deteriorating. The thymus gland produces hormones that may be responsible for keeping our immune system intact, as well as stimulating and controlling the production of neurotransmitters, which are chemical messengers that serve as the go-betweens among nerve cells.

Time also brings with it subtle body changes that may confuse your immune system. That confusion results in the body's production of antibodies against itself, since it believes its own cells to be a threat to your well-being. In essence, aging increases the chances that the body will turn against itself and destroy its own tissues. Autoimmune diseases such as rheumatoid arthritis or lupus may be the result.

MENTAL CHANGES

As you can imagine, it's impossible to study how any individual's brain reacts to time, but there are some general assumptions about what happens to brain tissue with age.

Although no one knows for sure why, the brain gets smaller with time, probably due to a decrease in fluid as well as neuron loss. Neurons are the nerve cells that make up most of the brain. You're born with upwards of 200 billion. Neurons communicate with each other via neurotransmitters, the body's chemical messengers.

In addition to fewer cells and less fluid in the brain, blood flow to the brain decreases by 15 to 20 percent from ages 30 to 70. Although there is less blood going to the brain and a moderate loss of brain tissue in healthy older people, the news isn't all bad. Despite the loss of cells, the cerebral cortex is remarkably intact, even well into the later years. That's most gratifying, since the cortex houses long-term memory and language skills, and it's the part of the brain most responsible for processing information and for creative thinking.

EXERCISE YOUR ACUMEN

If new situations make you squirm, maybe you should exercise more often. What's the connection? As you age, it takes more time for your brain to process new information, so you may avoid unfamiliar surroundings for the sake of comfort. But that just limits your world.

Regular exercise can help you expand your horizons. Studies show that the most physically fit older people best tolerate unfamiliar surroundings. Physical fitness helps you react more quickly to new situations, new faces, or a new social setting, perhaps adapting as quickly as someone much younger.

METABOLIC CHANGES

As you get older, it's normal to gain weight, right? It may be normal—if you define "normal" as "common"—but it's not desirable, and it's not inevitable either.

Chances are, you weigh more now than you did ten years ago. Or maybe your waistline has expanded, even as the scale has remained steady. Understanding what happens with weight as your body ages will help you to control it.

Beginning around age 25, total body fat starts to increase, while muscle mass and body water decrease. As a result, you may weigh more as you age or lose some of your muscle tone.

Why has your shape gone south? A lower basal metabolic rate (BMR) is to blame. BMR is the number of calories you burn daily to fuel involuntary body functions, such as your heartbeat, brain function, and digestion. BMR is dependent upon body composition. The more muscle you have, the more calories you burn, 24 hours a day. That's because muscle is a high-maintenance tissue and requires more calories than fat to sustain itself.

The decline in muscle mass that begins in your twenties, coupled with a decrease in activity level, means that you need fewer calories in your sixties than you did in your teens. For example, a 180-pound male's BMR accounts for about 1,930 calories a day between the ages of 18 and 30. After age 60, his body needs about 350 fewer calories to maintain his weight and good health. If you're still eating like a teenager by the time you're 60, and you haven't increased your physical activity, you'll definitely be putting on pounds.

For women, menopause often means weight gain. When the ovaries stop producing the hormone estrogen, muscle mass may diminish to the point of lowering BMR. When that happens, women gain a significant amount of fat, usually in the abdomen, even without consuming more calories.

Speaking of the abdomen, where you store extra fat also affects your health. If you're shaped like an apple—packing fat in your mid-section—you're at greater risk for heart disease than if you're shaped like a pear—gaining weight around your hips and buttocks. Excess weight in any location also boosts your chances for developing certain cancers and diabetes, and it also aggravates arthritis in your hips and knees.

As you age, your ability to maintain a normal level of glucose in your blood declines, raising the risk for type 2 diabetes. Glucose is the energy derived from food and is the fuel for cells. Glucose needs the hormone insulin, which is produced in your pancreas, to enter cells. Glucose intolerance means glucose roams free in the body, where high levels wreak havoc on blood vessels.

There are several reasons why glucose intolerance increases with age. You could have too much blood glucose because you don't export enough insulin from your pancreas to assist in the delivery of glucose to cells, your liver may make too much glucose (the liver is a reservoir of energy, albeit limited), or insulin fails to bind properly with your cells to allow it to escort glucose inside. Being overweight and inactive can lead to the latter.

The result of glucose intolerance, if not nipped in the bud, is diabetes.

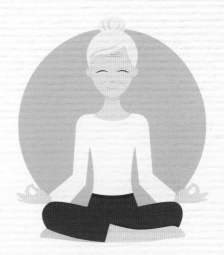

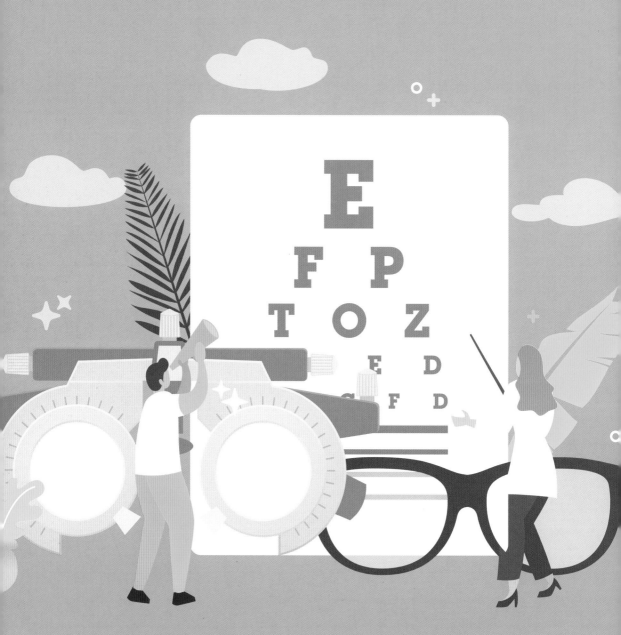

RESPIRATORY CHANGES

As you age, your lungs become less elastic, and your chest wall stiffens. In addition, the expansion of your trachea contributes to a decreased surface area in your lungs. You can't cough as forcefully, which also diminishes your ability to clear germs from your lungs. That's why older people are more prone to upper respiratory infections, such as colds. If you ever smoked, your respiratory potential is reduced in your later years. Older adults also experience some difficulties with swallowing, which increases the chances of aspirating particles of food or other substances into the lungs. Aspiration is a common cause of pneumonia in older adults.

Lung capacity and function drop off with time, which means you may be more winded after climbing a flight of stairs or taking a walk than you were 20 years ago, but exercise heads off some of the changes to the lungs and entire respiratory system. Physically active older people who regularly participate in aerobic exercises, including walking and cycling, are way ahead of the curve. Their aerobic capacity is far greater than their peers who don't exercise, and better than younger, sedentary people. In fact, well-conditioned older people may reach levels of lung function that exceed those of much younger people. A generous intake of vitamin C also helps maintain pulmonary function as you age. Loss of pulmonary function is a major predictor of disease and death in older adults.

EYESIGHT

Are you holding your newspaper at arm's length? Squinting at documents to see the fine print? Do you need more light to see clearly? Each passing decade brings changes that weaken eyesight, including the slow loss of ability to focus on close objects or small print. Presbyopia, the most common reason why you and your peers need reading glasses, is characterized by decreasing ability to focus on nearby objects. This condition typically shows up around age 40 but often develops for decades before that.

Some of the age-related eye changes are obvious, while others go undetected until vision is limited in some way. For example, the tissues surrounding eyes lose their tone, and fat is lost, too, which results in droopy upper eyelids and the turning outward or inward of the lower lid. On the other hand, cataracts, which cloud your vision by keeping the light from getting through the clear lens of the eye, are barely detectable because they form at a

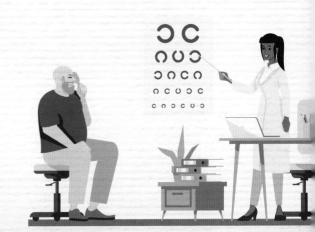

snail's pace, are painless, and don't result in any redness or tearing in the eye. Over the years, the iris, the colored part of your eyeball, loses flexibility. Your pupils—the black holes in the iris that respond to light—get smaller, and the lenses start to accumulate yellow substances, possibly as a result of exposure to sunlight. These changes predispose you to glaucoma, the product of excessive pressure inside your eyeball, which can lead to vision loss and blindness. No one knows the cause of glaucoma, but it is more prevalent in older people, African-Americans, and in those with a family history of the disease.

Glaucoma is basically symptom-free, often until it is too late. That's why the Glaucoma Research Foundation recommends testing for glaucoma every two to four years before age 40, every one to three years through age 54, every one to two years through age 65, and yearly after that. Get tested more frequently if you have risk factors such as:

- you have had eye injuries

- you have high blood pressure

- you've been using cortisone long-term

Decreased blood flow to the retina, the paper-thin tissue lining the back of your eyeball, can lead to macular degeneration. Macular degeneration destroys sharp, central vision.

HEARING

Do you find yourself saying "what?" more often? Maybe you don't like crowds as much since you can't detect the nuances of conversations that well. Hearing loss is one of the most common complaints of getting older, especially for men, who are more prone to hearing loss at any age.

Aging produces a progressive hearing loss at all frequencies, known as presbycusis. After age 55, your ability to detect changes in the pitch of sounds drops off dramatically, which can make your speech less understandable to others.

In addition, the walls of your ear canal thin out, and ear wax production falters. Your eardrum thickens. You may even get arthritis in the joints that connect the bones found in the inner ear. Yet, no one knows for sure if these changes in hearing can be put down to the aging process. But it's certain that the loss of hair cells is what diminishes hearing the most. Hair cells are part of the inner ear that help transmit impulses to a nerve that transfers them to your brain for processing. Nerve damage, injury, exposure to loud noise, and certain medications can cause hair cell loss.

Diminished hearing can isolate you from friends and family and limit your social involvement and enjoyment of life. Here are some questions developed by The National Institute on Deafness and Other

SCREENING SOLUTIONS

Many of the conditions affecting your aging eyes are detectable and treatable, allowing you to see clearly into a ripe old age. Some, such as cataracts and glaucoma, may be headed off by wearing sturdy sunglasses to protect eyes from sunlight. The irony is that not enough people are screened for the conditions that hamper vision.

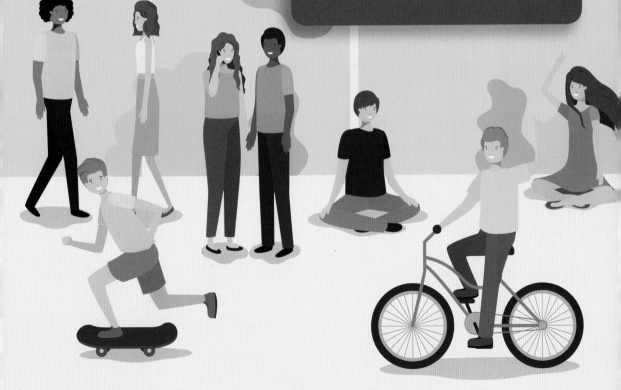

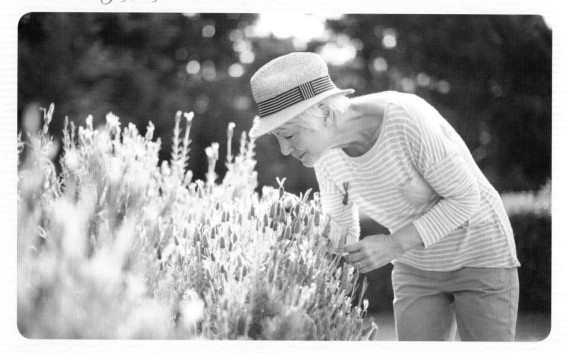

Communication Disorders to help you take stock of your hearing.

- Do you have a problem hearing over the telephone?

- Do you have trouble following the conversation when two or more people are talking at the same time?

- Do people complain that you turn the volume of the radio or television up too high?

- Do you have to strain to understand conversation?

- Do you have trouble hearing in a noisy background?

- Do you find yourself asking people to repeat themselves?

- Do many people you talk to seem to mumble or not speak clearly?

- Do you misunderstand what others are saying and respond inappropriately?

- Do you have trouble understanding the speech of women and children?

- Do people get annoyed because you misunderstand what they say?

Answering "Yes" to three or more of the above questions means you need to discuss your hearing loss with your doctor.

SMELL AND TASTE

You can thank your nose for your sense of taste, despite the thousands of taste buds populating your tongue: They can only detect a mere four out of thousands of possible flavors in foods.

The tongue recognizes only sweet, salty, bitter, and sour tastes. That's why enjoying food is limited without a healthy sense of smell. When you chew food and drink beverages, their aromas are released in your mouth. Saliva dissolves flavor-producing substances in food and drink that make contact with your tongue's taste buds. More importantly, dissolved flavor compounds waft up the back of your throat, making their way to receptor cells in your nose. From there, nerves transmit flavor messages to the brain, allowing you to perceive and enjoy them.

If you're having trouble savoring the flavor of food, blame it on a lessened sense of smell. Time dulls your sense of smell, but not usually until you reach age 60, and then it varies from person to person. About half of adults over the age of 65 suffer from some diminished sense of smell. On the other hand, your sense of taste for sweet, salty, bitter, and sour foods may be remarkably intact until you're well into your seventies.

A zinc deficiency can also cause a decreased sense of taste. Zinc supplementation can help restore it if you do have a deficiency.

Infections threaten sense of smell and, as a result, your ability to enjoy food. Some of the damage from the flu, colds, or hepatitis can be permanent. More often than not, acute illnesses, including sinus infections and seasonal allergies, block aromas from the receptor cells that relay flavor information to the brain. As a result, you don't have as much capacity to savor the flavors of food.

The pills you take every day to control medical conditions such as high blood pressure and arthritis can affect sense of taste, mainly by affecting the areas of the brain where you perceive flavors. Chemotherapy drugs and head and neck radiation also threaten flavor perception, sometimes permanently.

If you're eating more, but enjoying food less, you may be experiencing a diminished sense of smell or taste. Make the most of what you have with these eating tips.

- **Stay well.** Healthy seniors show less of a decline in their sense of smell and taste over time, compared with those who get sick more often. Boost your immune system with a well-balanced diet, regular exercise, and plenty of rest. Get a yearly flu shot.

- **Mind your medications.** Ask your pharmacist if the drugs you're taking could be disturbing your sense of taste and smell. Seek alternatives.

- **Cool it.** Avoid very hot foods and fluids. They can damage your taste buds.

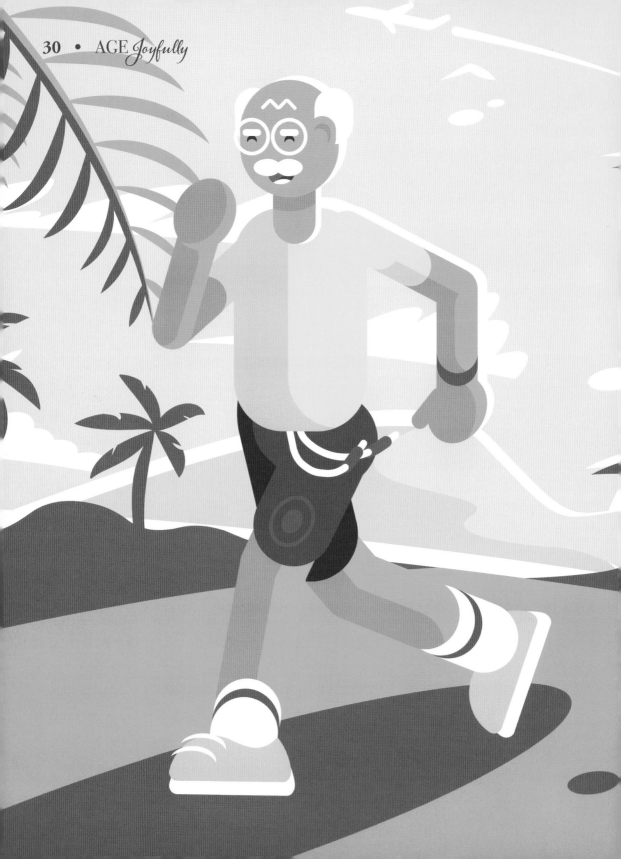

- **Keep them separated.** Switch often from one food to another during a meal, since successive bites of the same food decrease its perceived flavor. Avoid combining foods in your mouth, because it masks individual flavors and aromas.

- **Spice it up.** Season foods with herbs and spices and flavor-packed ingredients such as onions and garlic.

- **Slow down, you chew too fast.** Avoid gulping your food—you'll miss out on its taste. Make the flavor last by letting foods linger on your tongue.

- **Compensate.** When your sense of taste goes south, vary the temperature, texture, and colors of foods to capitalize on other aspects of eating enjoyment.

- **Quit smoking.** Cigarette smoking damages taste buds, blunting the taste of food.

- **Check it out.** If you have a sudden, inexplicable loss of taste or smell, or if you experience a persistent decline in either of these two senses, see your doctor to rule out the possibility of serious illness.

HYDRATION

No one gives much thought to the body's water balance, but it rules your life. All of the body's reactions that keep you alive would cease without adequate fluid. When you don't drink fluid, your body's balance is off-kilter. Yet, this vital nutrient is often given short shrift.

Problem is, by the time you get thirsty, you're already dehydrated. Your body may have lost up to two percent of its weight before it signals you to drink. That loss can impair your reasoning and judgment, as well as bodily functions. For example, dehydrated people can become easily confused. As you age, it gets harder for your body to activate its thirst mechanism to help you get the fluid you need.

You may try to avoid fluids if you're having trouble with incontinence, yet doing so can land you in the hospital as a result of dehydration, which is quite serious. Hyperthermia, or heatstroke, may be one result of not drinking enough when you're older. Hyperthermia happens when the body gets overheated, and it can be deadly if not treated immediately. It's more common with age, as your body cannot regulate its internal temperature with the efficiency of your youth. The symptoms of hyperthermia include headache, nausea, and fatigue, especially in hot humid weather or after being exposed to any heat, such as a warm, enclosed space.

HEAT AND COLD

Not too hot, not too cold? As we age, we lose some of our ability to regulate body temperature. A room that has a twenty-year-old running for a heavy sweater or sweating buckets may feel perfectly comfortable to a grandparent. Physical changes discussed earlier, such as loss of muscle, as well as reduced energy production, are partially responsible for decreased perception of cold. In addition, blood vessels in the skin do not have the same youthful ability to constrict in order to conserve heat, and you may not be able to shiver, which is heat-producing. Older people also lack the ability to dissipate normal body heat, and because of a decreased sense of thirst, they are more likely to be suffering from a lack of fluid. Thyroid disease, which is increasingly prevalent in older adults, can also be responsible for thermal insensitivity.

All these changes make older people more susceptible to both hypothermia, a condition in which body temperature dips below 96°F, and heatstroke. Both conditions are life-threatening. People age 75 and older are five times more likely to die of hypothermia than young people. Symptoms of hypothermia include sleepiness or confusion; leg or arm stiffness; slow, slurred speech; and low pulse rate. Heatstroke is fatal for ten percent of older people who experience it. Symptoms of heatstroke include high temperature, changes in mental function, and rapid heart rate and breathing.

REPRODUCTIVE FUNCTION

Most of your organs get smaller with age, but the prostate gets bigger. With time, there is a decline in blood flow, and prostate tissue is replaced with scar tissue. A bigger prostate gland may be the result of decreased concentrations of testosterone.

The prostate is normally about the size of a small egg. It's located below the bladder, wrapping around the urethra, which is the tube that carries urine from the bladder. The prostate makes a fluid that becomes part of semen, which transports sperm. Prostate problems are common in men age 50 and older. More than half of all men in their sixties suffer from benign prostatic hyperplasia (BPH), the enlargement of the prostate.

The average age of menopause is 51 in the United States, although it can occur up to age 55. The changes that menopause brings can be obvious well before a woman stops menstruating. Estrogen produced in the ovaries is significantly reduced with menopause. In turn, many women complain of hot flashes and experience changes in the uterus and vagina. The uterine lining and the tissue lining the vagina gets thinner, connective tissue proliferates, and vaginal secretions decrease, all of which can make sexual intercourse painful. Lack of estrogen also increases problems with urinary incontinence. You may notice more cysts in your breasts, as well.

A SUMMARY OF SOLUTIONS

While the list of changes that come with aging isn't a fun read, it can be empowering. When you know the potential issues that come with aging, you can forestall many of them. Here are four simple steps you can take to help your health and keep your system in good shape.

EXERCISE has been mentioned several times in this chapter, because it helps in so many different ways, both physically and mentally. *Aerobic exercise* that gets your heart pumping helps your cardiovascular system and pulmonary function. *Weight-bearing exercise*—and something as simple as walking is a weight-bearing exercise—helps your muscles and bones. Building activity into your life may be the best way to reverse aging. It provides benefits across the board.

GET SCREENED. The sooner you know about some problems, the sooner they can be addressed. Make it a practice to get regularly screened for silent issues that can creep up on you. Specifically, get regularly screened for high blood pressure, high glucose levels, high cholesterol, and vision problems.

STAY HYDRATED. Get in the habit of drinking water regularly, even if you don't feel thirsty. Fruit such as melons and citrus fruit can also help you stay hydrated.

EAT LESS FOOD WITH MORE NUTRIENTS. Being overweight can affect cardiovascular health, as well as joint and muscle health. As we get older, our body's ability to absorb certain crucial nutrients can decline, so it's important to make sure we're getting enough of those. In the next chapter, we'll specifically discuss food and the changes you can make to your diet to optimize your health.

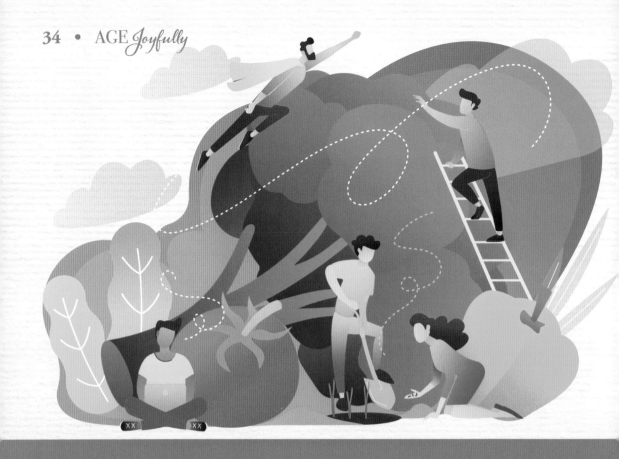

YOUR CHANGING NUTRITIONAL NEEDS

As you get older, you need more of some nutrients and less of others to accommodate—or delay—age-related body changes. In fact, a nutrient-rich diet can head off slow, insidious nutrient deficiencies that can have a considerable impact on your well-being. Nutrient inadequacies often go undetected and can mimic the effects of aging. Even borderline deficiencies in vitamin B12, for instance, can cause memory loss and other symptoms that are often mistaken for senility.

The nutritional picture is complicated by the fact that your calorie needs actually decrease as you get older. That means you have to pack more nutrition into less food. If your diet was already deficient in some vitamins and minerals, it will only become more so unless you make good food choices. Your body changes also affect the way you process medications, including the way in which food and medications interact.

INCREASING NEEDS

There are many more nutrients for which your needs increase as you get older than those for which they decrease. For some nutrients, such as vitamin D and calcium, the actual amount you need to consume every day goes up. For other nutrients, such as vitamin B12, the recommended daily intake doesn't increase, but getting the right amount becomes both increasingly important and increasingly difficult because of age-related body changes. So different are the nutritional needs of older adults that Tufts University, with support from the AARP Foundation, put out a My Plate for Older Adults in 2016 to emphasize the nutritional needs of seniors. (See https://hnrca. tufts.edu/myplate/)

THE B VITAMINS

The B vitamins are a tight group. Their functions are similar, and they are closely related, often depending on each other and working together toward good health.

Energy production is the primary function of the B vitamins. But these water-soluble vitamins also are important for other biological functions, such as homocysteine metabolism. While all the B vitamins are important in aging, those mentioned here play a particular role in tempering the changes that your body faces with advancing time.

RIBOFLAVIN

Without riboflavin, you can't harness the energy from the calories that food provides. Riboflavin assists your body's energy production in all of its cells, and it's critical to vision and skin health. It may help protect your eyes by curtailing cataract formation. In addition, riboflavin helps transform the amino acid tryptophan into niacin, another B vitamin involved in the body's metabolism that also plays a role in its use of fat.

While calorie needs drop off with time, riboflavin requirements remain constant. That's why a 75-year-old needs just as much riboflavin as a 19-year-old: Females need 1.1 milligrams (mg) of riboflavin daily; men need 1.3 mg. Riboflavin requirements are linked to general body size and the number of calories you eat, which is why the requirements for men are higher than for women. Experts suspect that the older you get, the more sensitive you are to riboflavin deficiencies, which is a good reason for consuming the recommended daily amount.

Regular strenuous physical activity may boost riboflavin requirements, regardless of age. If you're working out more to arrest the muscle tissue loss that's associated with aging, you may need extra riboflavin. Taking a multivitamin that provides 100 percent of the RDA for vitamin B2 should ensure sufficient riboflavin intake.

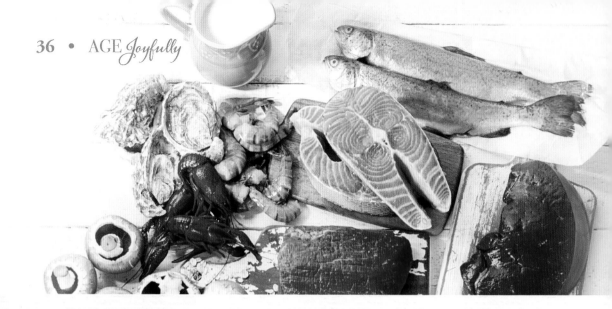

Riboflavin intake among most Americans has generally been found to be adequate, as long as you don't live on highly processed foods. That's probably because riboflavin is found in a wide array of foods, including milk (buy brands in cardboard cartons or opaque plastic containers, since they preserve light-sensitive riboflavin), yogurt, enriched breads and grains, and organ meats such as beef liver. Other sources of riboflavin include green vegetables and eggs.

However, up to 36 percent of older adults are not getting 100 percent of the RDA for riboflavin through their diets. Vegetarians and vegans are more likely to have issues with riboflavin intake.

VITAMIN B6

Vitamin B6 is essential to new cell growth. Along with riboflavin, vitamin B6 helps transform the amino acid tryptophan to niacin, another B vitamin responsible for energy production and use. Vitamin B6 also participates in the process that converts tryptophan to the neurotransmitter serotonin, a chemical messenger that fosters brain-cell communication.

Vitamin B6 boosts the immune system while keeping blood glucose levels in check. Along with vitamin B12 and the B vitamin folate, vitamin B6 may help decrease homocysteine levels in the bloodstream. Since high homocysteine concentrations have been linked to increased heart disease and stroke risk, vitamin B6 is believed to help ward off those life-threatening conditions.

The older you get, the greater the risk of vitamin B6 deficiencies, according to government consumption studies. There are two reasons for this. Since vitamin B6 and protein occur together naturally in foods, people who don't consume enough protein—which is most common among older adults—

will also be deficient in vitamin B6. Also, some research suggests that vitamin B6 requirements increase with age because of an increased metabolism of the compound. While the recommended daily intake for adults up to age 50 is 1.3 milligrams (mg) for both men and women, the RDA for people over 50 increases to 1.7 milligrams (mg) for men and 1.5 milligrams (mg) for women. And if you don't get enough vitamin B6, you're probably low in most other B vitamins, too.

Skin problems, anemia, depression, confusion, and even convulsions can occur without adequate vitamin B6. And, since vitamin B6 helps regulate blood sugar, a deficiency in it may boost blood glucose levels as well as levels of insulin. Excessive blood glucose damages blood vessels and often leads to organ destruction. Kidneys and eyes are particularly vulnerable. Studies show that taking extra vitamin B6 may help improve age-related declines in memory.

Vitamin B6 beefs up immunity, which typically wanes with age. It does this by boosting production of white blood cells and antibodies, which fend off bacteria, viruses, fungi, and parasites. Vitamin B6 also helps your body seek out and destroy the cell proliferation that can give rise to cancerous tumors.

Poultry and fish are rich in vitamin B6, along with potatoes and non-citrus fruit.

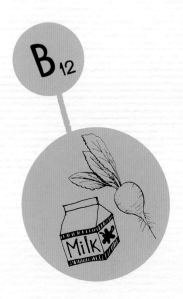

VITAMIN B12

Vitamin B12 is essential for normal neurologic function and red blood cell formation as well as for fat metabolism. So important is B12 to mental functioning that even borderline deficiencies in it can cause memory loss and other symptoms that mimic dementia. Deficiencies can also cause difficulties with balance, muscle coordination, and manual dexterity. Studies show that people with low blood levels of vitamin B12 do not have the same spatial relationship skills of those with higher B12 concentrations. Vitamin B12 deficiencies can cause serious damage to the nervous system, which is irreversible if the condition persists for long.

Heading off heart disease, stroke, and peripheral vascular disease—a condition that

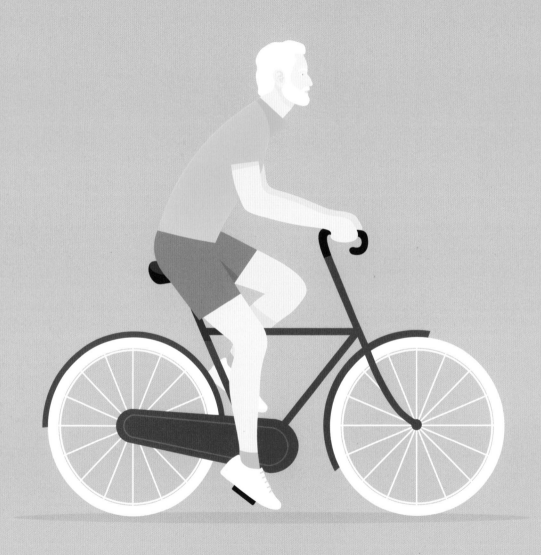

curtails circulation in your extremities—is another important vitamin B12 function. The vitamin works with two other B vitamins, folate and vitamin B6, to lower homocysteine concentrations in the bloodstream, thus helping prevent these life-threatening diseases. A vitamin B12 deficiency due to a lack of intrinsic factor, a substance made in the stomach, can cause pernicious anemia. Vitamin B12 injections are necessary when intrinsic factor is lacking.

Although your need for vitamin B12 doesn't increase with age (it remains at 2.4 micrograms daily), your ability to absorb enough of this important vitamin may be compromised, necessitating supplementation. That's because as many as 30 percent of people age 50 and older (and 40 percent of those age 80 and older) have atrophic gastritis, a condition in which the body does not produce enough stomach acid to allow absorption of vitamin B12 from foods. Most people never realize they have this condition.

Since synthetic vitamin B12 doesn't require stomach acid, make sure you get sufficient quantities of it through supplements or from fortified foods, such as breakfast cereals. Even if you don't have atrophic gastritis, supplementation of up to 100 percent of the RDA probably won't hurt you. Considering the health consequences of a deficiency, it's better to be safe.

Aside from fortified foods, beef liver and clams are two of the most concentrated sources of vitamin B12. But fish, meat, poultry, eggs, and many dairy products are also good sources.

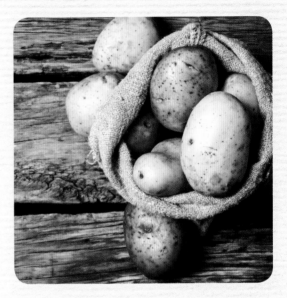

FOLATE/FOLIC ACID

Folate is the naturally occurring variety of a B vitamin found in foods such as legumes, spinach, and orange juice. Folic acid, its synthetic sibling, is added to vitamin pills and to products made from enriched flour, such as bread. Folate is the umbrella term often used to refer to all of the forms of this important B vitamin, and it is the term that will be used in this chapter.

Getting enough folate becomes increasingly important as you age because of its role in the prevention of heart attack, stroke, and circulation problems. Along with vitamins B6 and B12, folate helps rid your bloodstream of excess homocysteine, an amino acid that fosters clogged arteries, blocking the flow of blood to your brain, heart, and extremities. Age boosts homocysteine concentrations in your blood. Research shows that men and women under age 60 with the highest homocysteine levels run the greatest risk of heart disease and circulation problems.

Although the recommended intake of folate remains at 400 micrograms for adults age 51 or older, the vast majority of older adults fall far short of the requirement. Approximately three out of four adults get less than the recommended amount, putting them at risk not just for heart disease but also for megaloblastic anemia, cancer, and depression.

Folate prevents a type of blood disorder known as megaloblastic anemia by facilitating DNA replication within healthy red blood cells that transport oxygen to working cells. The DNA must replicate before the cell can divide. If it can't divide, the cell becomes enlarged, or megaloblastic. Folate may also protect against certain cancers, particularly those of the cervix, colon, and rectum. It's not known exactly how folate is linked to a lower incidence of these cancers, but it seems that a folate deficiency may push your body over the edge if you're prone to developing these types of cancer.

Without adequate folate, protein production falters, affecting the growth and repair of tissues, which you want to keep in top form as the years go by. While the effects are most noticeable during periods of rapid growth, including infancy and adolescence, a folate shortfall shouldn't be ignored, no matter what your age. As you get older, your cells need all the help they can get to maintain themselves and to replicate in a healthy manner, so that tissues and organs function optimally.

Researchers strongly suspect that this B vitamin is linked to mental health, particularly in seniors. Folate may help prevent depression and preserve mental acumen.

Try to meet your daily requirement with a combination of vitamin supplements, fortified foods, and a folate-rich diet. In the case of folate, manmade sources are often better than natural sources because your body absorbs the synthetic form of the vitamin almost twice as efficiently. Folate-rich foods are important to your health, however, and you should still try to eat plenty of plant-based foods. Green vegetables are especially important in order to get enough folate: the NIH recommends spinach, asparagus, and mustard greens. Nuts, peas, and beans also provide folate.

CHOLINE

You may not have heard of choline, but this B-like vitamin has been officially recognized as an essential nutrient by the Food and Nutrition Board (FNB) of the National Academy of Science's Institute of Medicine.

So what is choline good for? It serves as the raw material for several substances in the body, including the neurotransmitter acetylcholine, a chemical messenger that ferries information between brain cells and is involved in muscle control. Animal studies show that consuming adequate choline early in life leads to a reduction in the seriousness of memory deficits, such as dementia, when you are older. Of course, the earlier you begin eating a healthy diet based on balance, variety, and moderation, the greater your chances of staying sharp later on.

Choline is the raw material of cell membranes—the wrappers around cells that preserve their integrity and strength. In addition, choline is vital to liver health and may help your body clear excessive levels of homocysteine, an amino acid that initiates the clogging of arteries, from your bloodstream.

The FNB sets requirements at 550 milligrams (mg) of choline every day for males age 51 and older and 425 mg for females in that age group. Experts have hinted at an increasing need for choline among older adults but have not set a higher recommended intake for them.

Choline recommendations have limited value, however, because you can't find choline counts on the Nutrition Facts label on food products or in most nutrient databases, no matter how expansive. No reliable figures for the choline content of foods exist right now. That said, there are some ways to boost choline intake. Experts say that milk, eggs, beef, and peanuts head up the list of the richest choline sources. Your best bet for meeting your daily requirement of choline is to eat a wide array of foods, since choline is found to some extent in many different types of foods, including potatoes, whole grains, cauliflower, Brussels sprouts, and broccoli.

VITAMIN C

There's more to vitamin C than cold prevention. True, vitamin C is vital for forming the white blood cells that fight infection, including the common cold virus, and other diseases, such as cancer. But vitamin C can't prevent colds all by itself; it takes an otherwise robust immune system. What's more, its duties transcend bolstering the immune system.

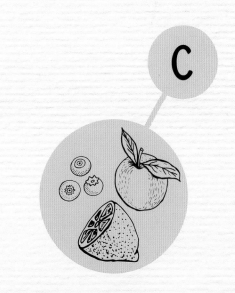

This water-soluble vitamin is involved in the production of collagen, which could be called your body's cement. Collagen is a connective tissue that provides structure by keeping skin taut, muscles firm, and bones dense, among other duties. Vitamin C bolsters blood vessel wall strength and keeps intact tiny blood vessels, such as capillaries, which helps prevent bruising.

But vitamin C doesn't stop there. It's also responsible for red blood cell formation, wound healing, and healthy gums. And best of all, vitamin C is an antioxidant, helping to neutralize destructive forms of oxygen known as free radicals, which damage DNA and turn normal cells into cancerous monsters.

The recommended intake of vitamin C for adults is 90 milligrams (mg) each day for men and 75 mg for women. Smokers require at least 35 mg more than that per day, since smoking decreases vitamin C in your bloodstream and soft tissues. Getting adequate amounts of vitamin C every day is important because most of the vitamin isn't stored in the body beyond 24 hours.

Vitamin C's potent antioxidant abilities are particularly important as you get older because they help stave off diseases that are more common with age, including the following:

- **HEART DISEASE.** Vitamin C could stall heart disease in older people, possibly by increasing blood levels of high density lipoproteins (HDL, or the "good" cholesterol) while suppressing low density lipoproteins (LDL, or the "bad" cholesterol). LDL cholesterol is the kind that sticks to artery walls, clogging the blood vessels and restricting blood flow. Vitamin C may also reduce the risk of developing high blood pressure or help control it in seniors.

- **CATARACTS AND MACULAR DEGENERATION.** Free radicals can oxidize the cells of the lens in your eyes, leading to cataracts, which are common with increasing age. While it seems that eye damage is inevitable, the body employs a sophisticated system to repel free radicals, but unfortunately, that mechanism

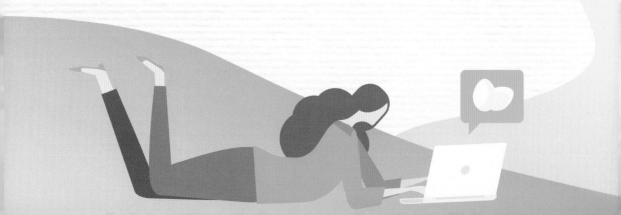

wanes with time. Studies show that high vitamin C intake is associated with a decreased chance of developing cataracts and macular degeneration, which is also related to aging. Vitamin C is so effective at preserving vision that eating less than the recommended daily amount may actually promote cataract formation.

◆ **CANCER.** Vitamin C's antioxidant powers are also responsible for its ability to fight cancer. Cancer risk increases with age, so it makes sense to bolster vitamin C intake. Vitamin C can probably help protect you against certain cancers, including those of the esophagus, stomach, and pancreas, and may also ward off cervical, rectal, breast, and lung cancers.

◆ **ANEMIA.** Vitamin C also enhances the absorption of iron from foods, which is particularly helpful to premenopausal women, who still require iron to replenish monthly blood losses.

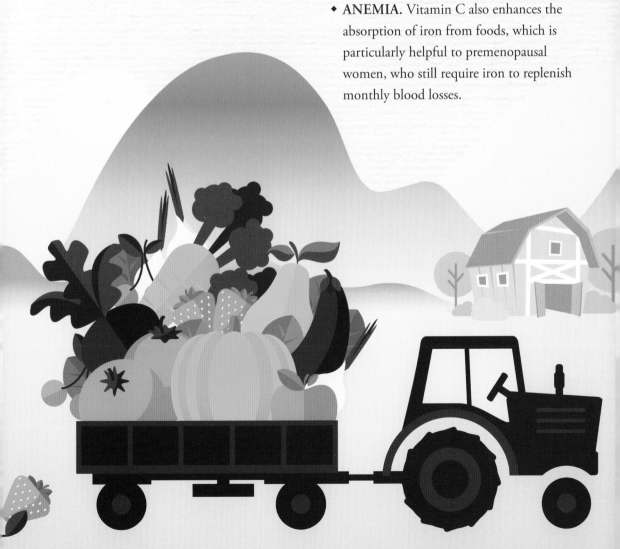

Citrus fruits and tomatoes are common sources of vitamin C. It is also found in red and green bell peppers, baked potatoes, and cantaloupe.

VITAMIN D

Vitamin D is critical to bone health and strength. Think of it as a bank teller that facilitates the deposits and withdrawals of calcium from your bone "bank account." Since you need a certain amount of calcium in your bloodstream at all times for survival, vitamin D stands at the ready, 24 hours a day, to make sure calcium is available to your cells. When you consume calcium, vitamin D ensures that it gets safely into your skeletal storehouse.

As you age, you have an increasing need for vitamin D. When you're over 70, the recommended daily intake for adults goes from 600 international units (IU) to 800 IU. If you have kidney or liver disease, you may need even more because those organs help convert vitamin D to its active form. In fact, the vitamin is stored in the liver for later use.

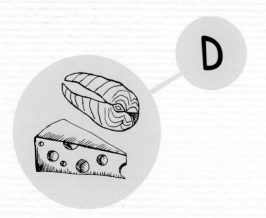

Why such a change in requirements? Because your skin, which converts sunlight into vitamin D, is not as effective at the conversion process as you age. Not only do you make less vitamin D, you don't absorb it as well from foods. And if you don't get out much, and you wear sunscreen when you are outside, you are at particular risk for vitamin D deficiency due to lack of sunlight. That's why you may need a vitamin D supplement, especially if you're over 70.

Research has revealed that consuming vitamin D along with calcium at any time of your life makes a difference in your risk for bone fracture—even in your eighties. It may even help you build bone after menopause, when bone tissue is lost at a good clip.

In its natural state, food is a relatively poor source of vitamin D. Vitamin D is added to nearly all milk in the United States, however. One glass provides 100 IU. But adults tend to shy away from milk, thinking it is kids' stuff. The lack of vitamin-D–rich food sources and sunlight is probably one of the reasons why studies suggest that up to 40 percent of adults over the age of 50 have borderline vitamin D deficiencies and don't even know it. Vitamin D supplements can help you achieve an adequate intake.

Some of the better food sources for vitamin D includes salmon and tuna, beef liver, eggs, and mushrooms.

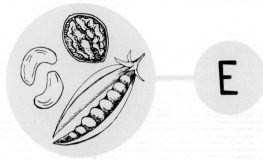

VITAMIN E

Like vitamin C, vitamin E functions as a cellular bodyguard, protecting the body's most basic units against the ravages of free radicals. When free radicals run rampant throughout your system, looking to snare an electron from a healthy cell, vitamin E readily donates one and spares cells from wholesale destruction.

Although the recommended daily intake of 22 international units (IU), or 15 milligrams (mg), for adults doesn't increase after age 50, surveys show that many Americans don't come close to meeting it. However, vitamin E's antioxidant properties make it one of your best defenses against a host of chronic conditions and illnesses that become more common as you age. These include heart disease, cataracts, and prostate cancer.

Vitamin E prevents the conversion of low density lipoprotein cholesterol (LDL, the "bad" cholesterol) to a more damaging form that leads to heart disease. And, because vitamin E makes blood more fluid, it reduces your risk of having clogged arteries or blood clots. Clots can restrict the flow of blood to the point of causing tissue death.

Vitamin E, along with vitamin C and beta-carotene, may delay the onset of cataracts or prevent cataract formation entirely. These antioxidants help fight the oxidation of the lens of the eye, which causes cataracts—one of the leading causes of blindness in older adults.

If you work out strenuously, expect to need more vitamin E. There is scientific evidence that prolonged exercise in seniors damages muscles and boosts conversion of LDL to a more damaging form. Older people who take large doses of supplemental vitamin E can avoid these detrimental effects to the point of being comparable to younger subjects.

Very large doses of 800 to 1,000 IU of vitamin E a day also appear to have a beneficial effect on those with Alzheimer disease. The risk of Alzheimer disease increases as you age, but studies suggest that vitamin E can delay some of its symptoms. There is no evidence, however, that similar amounts of vitamin E prevent the condition.

As if all of this isn't enough, as little as an extra 50 IU of vitamin E a day may help stave off prostate cancer.

Sources of vitamin E include some vegetable oils, particularly sunflower and safflower oil, nuts, particularly almonds, and seeds.

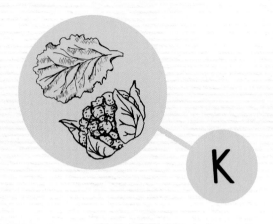

vitamin K, especially leafy green vegetables that are filled with other important nutrients. Blueberries, figs, and soybeans are also sources of vitamin K. There is a caveat, however. If you take any anticoagulant medications such as coumadin and heparin or consume aspirin or large doses of vitamin E supplements daily, ask your doctor first about increasing your vitamin K consumption. Since vitamin K promotes clotting, it could work against those anticoagulant medications.

VITAMIN K

As vitamins go, K lives in the shadows. You probably don't know that this obscure vitamin is made by bacteria in your intestine or that it helps blood to clot, preventing uncontrollable bleeding. And chances are, you don't even realize its role in keeping bones strong, helping to head off osteoporosis along with vitamin D, calcium, and a well-balanced diet.

The recommended dietary allowance (RDA) is 90 micrograms (mcg) for adult women and 120 mcg for adult men. However, research has also shown it takes at least 109 mcg of vitamin K a day to protect against hip fractures. That's the amount found in one-half cup cooked broccoli or in a little more than one-quarter cup cooked spinach. Since hip fractures are much more common with age, it won't hurt to eat more foods that are high in

CALCIUM

If it weren't for calcium, none of us would be standing up very straight. Calcium, the most abundant mineral in the body, builds and maintains strong bones and teeth. Nearly all the calcium in your body is stored in your skeleton, from which it is often called upon to regulate blood calcium concentrations— an absolute must for survival. Inadequate levels of calcium in your bloodstream have a detrimental effect on heart rhythm, muscle contraction and relaxation, and your ability to clot blood.

Calcium needs increase by about 200 milligrams (mg) a day after age 50 (women) or 70 (men), primarily to help prevent or minimize age-related bone loss. The Food and Nutrition Board (FNB) recommends a daily intake of 1,200 mg for women age 50 and older and men age 70 and older.

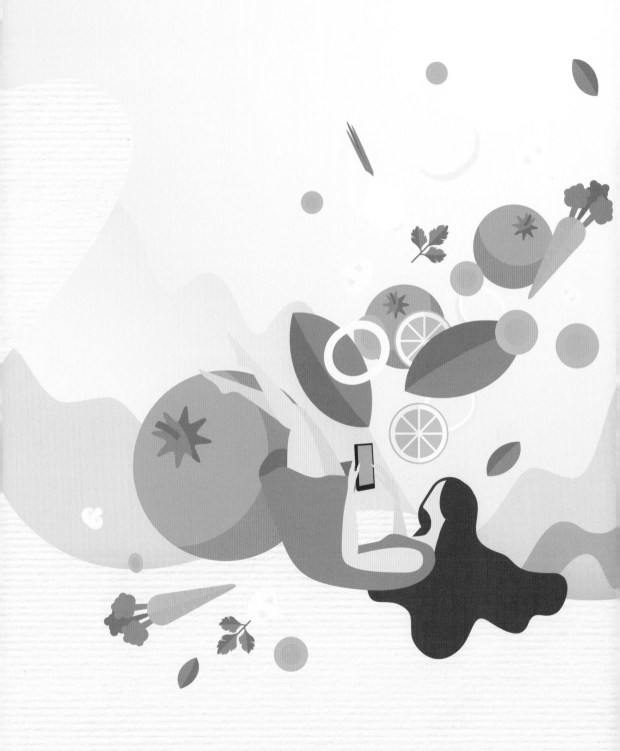

If you choose more calcium-rich food to meet the higher calcium recommendations, don't be concerned about overdoing it. The FNB says that you'd have to take about 2,000 mg of calcium or more every day for prolonged periods of time to cause kidney stones and high blood calcium and to hinder the uptake of the minerals iron, zinc, and magnesium by the body. You should, however, watch your intake of calcium via supplements, as it's not too difficult to get 2,000 mg that way.

There's been a lot of media attention to age-related bone loss and the importance of getting enough calcium through diet and supplementation. Still, research shows that most American adults consume less than half of the recommended daily intake. This is especially serious because, as your need for calcium increases, your body's ability to absorb it from foods decreases. In order to absorb calcium from food, you need a sufficient amount of stomach acid. But an estimated 30 percent of Americans over age 50 have atrophic gastritis, a condition in which the stomach does not produce enough acid. Most of these people are not aware that they have the condition, putting them at greater risk for osteoporosis.

Deficient calcium intake, coupled with a deficit in vitamin D—which is necessary for the body's absorption of calcium—causes the risk of fracture to skyrocket in older people. Several studies show that giving older people between 500 and 1,200 mg of calcium a day plus large doses of vitamin D (about 700 or 800 IU a day) slows bone loss and decreases the incidence of fractures.

What's more, calcium-rich diets may tame high blood pressure and put the kibosh on colon cancer. The Dietary Approaches to Stop Hypertension (DASH) study found that eating a low-fat diet (about 25 percent of calories) filled with fruits, vegetables, whole grain products, and two to three servings of calcium-laden low-fat or fat-free dairy products lowered blood pressure with the same success as medication. While researchers say that no one knows for sure exactly why the diet works, calcium most certainly plays a role along with several other nutrients.

Taking 1,200 mg of calcium daily also seemed to reduce the number of polyps (tumors that often turn into cancer) found in the colon.

Dairy products such as yogurt and milk are rich in calcium. Those who are lactose intolerant can seek out calcium in canned fish such as sardines and salmon, green vegetables, especially kale and broccoli, and products that are enriched with calcium. Some brands of orange or grape juice, for example, have a calcium-enriched version, and breakfast cereals may as well.

MAGNESIUM

Magnesium is essential for bone health. In fact, more than half the magnesium in your body is housed in your bones, lending strength to your skeleton. The remainder is deployed throughout your cells, participating in 300 or more body functions including muscle contraction, protein synthesis, cell reproduction, energy metabolism, and nutrient transport. In partnership with insulin, magnesium also helps control blood glucose levels. This mineral also keeps major blood vessels elastic and fluid and may curb high blood pressure. People who consume the most magnesium may be at lower risk for heart attack, too.

Technically, the recommended daily intake for magnesium doesn't increase with age. The recommended daily intake for men is 410–420 milligrams (mg), while the recommended intake for women is 310–320 milligrams. But magnesium is important in your later years, and studies show that we are eating less magnesium than ever. That's because unprocessed foods, particularly grains, are the richest sources, yet we're relying more and more on processed and convenience foods. Nuts and seeds are also good sources of magnesium, as well as legumes and green leafy vegetables.

Magnesium deficiencies can be caused by prolonged illness and poor diet, both of which tend to be more common in the later years. You're also at greater risk for magnesium deficiency if you have diabetes, a condition that also becomes increasingly common with age. People with diabetes may have low levels of magnesium in their cells, which may be the reason for elevated glucose concentrations in the blood, levels which tend to rise with age anyway.

Magnesium's ability to keep blood vessels supple is also increasingly important as you age since the risk of cardiovascular disease rises. Getting enough magnesium also protects against a fatally abnormal heartbeat, which could be the result of illness.

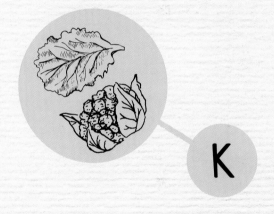

POTASSIUM

Potassium is in every cell in your body and is critical to normal muscle activity, nerve impulses, fluid balance, and normal blood pressure. Without it, you couldn't make a single move.

As you age, blood pressure often rises, and a potassium deficiency can be the culprit. A potassium deficiency is common, particularly as we consume more convenience and fast

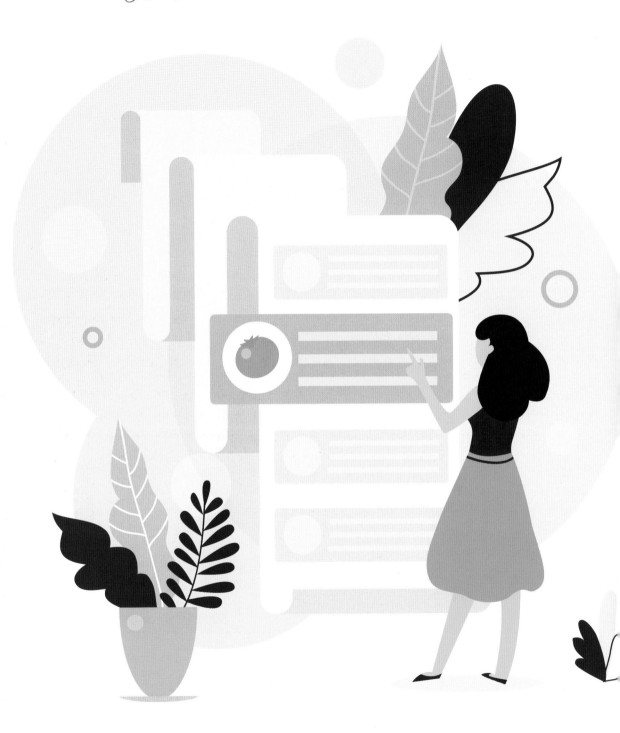

foods, which don't contain potassium, and less fruits, vegetables, and unprocessed grains, which contain the most potassium. A diet consisting primarily of processed foods will not provide sufficient potassium to drive down high blood pressure and to thwart its development. Potassium is also concentrated in dairy products, meat, fish, and poultry. The recommended daily intake for this mineral is 4,700 milligrams (mg).

If you do have high blood pressure and are taking medication for it, those very medications may be contributing to a potassium deficiency. Some high blood pressure medications cause your body to excrete potassium. If this is the case, you need even more of this mighty mineral.

Short- and long-term illness can affect your potassium supplies, especially when you've been avoiding food and drink, and even more so when you have been vomiting or had diarrhea for a few days. Since older people get sick more often, potassium's potential should not be overlooked.

Bananas are a prime source of potassium, as are certain dried fruits: apricots, prunes, and raisins. Potatoes, acorn squash, lentils, kidney beans, and nuts also provide potassium.

SELENIUM

Remember vitamin E, the antioxidant that thwarts cell damage caused by free radicals?

Well, the mineral selenium belongs to the same class of nutrient superheroes. It works with vitamin E to help protect cells. Much of selenium's power to fend off free radicals is the result of its ability to increase production of glutathione peroxidase, an enzyme produced by the body that is the paramount weapon in your body's sophisticated defense system. As an antioxidant, selenium helps protect against cancers of the colon, prostate, and lung and may pump up your immune system.

Getting the recommended daily intake—55 micrograms (mcg)—becomes increasingly important with age because your immune system gets weaker. That makes you prone to short- and long-term illness. Selenium may be able to help ward off myriad diseases as it boosts your immunity.

When it comes to cancer, risk increases with time, too, especially for the three cancers that selenium may be helpful in preventing: those of the prostate, lung, and colon.

Selenium is found in seafood and other animal products, as well as many grain products. Selenium in plant products depends on the soil in which they were grown.

CHROMIUM

Chromium helps your body keep blood glucose levels within normal range. It boosts the efficiency of the hormone insulin, promoting the uptake of glucose by the cells.

Chromium is also necessary for the metabolism of carbohydrate and fat and may reduce blood cholesterol and triglyceride (fat) concentrations.

As you get older, chromium concentrations decline in your body. That doesn't bode well for proper blood glucose control, since glucose concentrations creep up with age, wreaking havoc on blood vessels and resulting in organ damage. Chromium is so important to normal blood glucose levels that a deficiency is signaled by some of the same symptoms seen in diabetes, including an elevated blood glucose concentration; increased levels of triglycerides in the blood, which boost heart disease risk; and nerve damage in the extremities.

The RDA of chromium for people over 50 is 30 micrograms (mcg) for men and 20 mcg for women. While flat-out chromium deficits are rare in healthy adults, chronically low-chromium diets may not be—and that could be one reason that certain older individuals develop type 2 diabetes, as there is some evidence that people with type 2 diabetes are chromium deficient.

Chromium supplementation may sound like a simple solution, especially to someone with diabetes looking to decrease their medication dose. But there's no scientifically accurate way to measure chromium deficiency. Still, there's hope for some people with diabetes. In a scientific study, older adults with elevated glucose levels were able to normalize them when given chromium supplements.

Studies also show that chromium reduces heart disease risk by fostering lower levels of total blood cholesterol and triglycerides. Experts suspect that chromium supplementation produces such dramatic effects in people who are already deficient, however.

Meats and whole grain foods are standard sources of chromium.

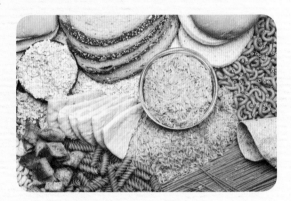

ZINC

Zinc is especially necessary for breaking down and using carbohydrate, fat, and protein. This mineral participates in the making of DNA, the cell's pattern for reproduction, and is considered crucial for the strength of cell membranes, the wrapper that protects the cell's inner workings. As part of insulin, zinc plays a role in normalizing blood glucose levels, helping to head off the damage done by excessive glucose in the blood vessels. Last, but not least, zinc bolsters immunity and wound healing and is necessary for a normal sense of taste. Whew!

Most older adults don't get enough zinc—experts have said that 90 percent of older Americans may take in suboptimal amounts of zinc. That may be especially true if you're avoiding fatty foods, such as red meat, in the name of heart health. Animal foods are packed with zinc.

Too little zinc has myriad implications for good health. Stresses, including physical trauma such as a broken bone, and wounds, including surgery, are more common with age, increasing your vulnerability to zinc deficiency. Older adults often have difficulty healing wounds, and it appears that zinc supplementation corrects slow wound healing in seniors, but only if they are deficient in zinc in the first place. Once zinc levels have returned to normal, extra zinc does not seem to speed up healing. Chronic blood loss, such as a bleeding ulcer, and conditions including diabetes and burns also boost zinc needs.

Immunity is especially vulnerable to zinc deficiencies. Without adequate zinc, your body is incapable of producing white blood cells to fight off infection as well as the antibodies you require to fend off invaders such as bacteria, viruses, fungi, and parasites and to squash mutant cells that can turn into cancerous tumors.

The RDA for zinc is 11 milligrams (mg) for men and 8 mg for women. A high zinc intake—over 60 milligrams a day—may suppress immune responsiveness and alter your sense of taste.

To eat more zinc, turn to the sea: oysters, lobsters, and crabs are great sources of zinc. Red meat and poultry also contain zinc in good quantities.

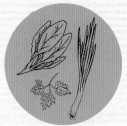

PROTEIN

When you were growing up, chances are most of your meals centered around meat. A nice juicy steak surrounded by a paltry portion of rice and, as a nod to the vegetable group, one or two stalks of limp broccoli were commonplace. Or maybe bacon and eggs were the stars of your morning meal, the supporting cast consisting of toast and juice. For many of us, protein-packed foods were front and center in our mothers' minds.

And with good reason, albeit to a certain extent. Foods such as meat, poultry, seafood, eggs, dairy products, nuts, and soy products are essential to life at any age because of the protein they pack. Protein helps:

- produce new cells, such as the antibodies that fight infection, repair tissues and organs, and generate genetic material.

- ferry cholesterol and fat around the body in fat/protein packages called lipoproteins.

- make enzymes, hormones, and the chemical messengers called neurotransmitters

- control fluid balance in your body.

The very notion of a daily protein requirement is misleading. What you really require are the amino acids that food protein provides. Your body needs 20 amino acids for good health. You can make 11 of them, but the balance, known as essential amino acids, must come from protein-packed foods. Amino acids found in food are no more vital than the amino acids your body puts out; they are called "essential" because your body cannot make them.

When you eat, digestion breaks down protein to amino acids. Your body reassembles these amino acids, as well as the ones it makes, into body parts and substances on an as-needed basis (which is 24 hours a day). Protein production is an exact science, and the unique pattern for each body protein is fixed. No deviations from the pattern are tolerated, and no substitutions are allowed in protein construction. That means if you are short just one amino acid, the production of a particular body protein comes to a halt. If this happens again and again, your health can suffer.

When your diet lacks calories, your body is signaled to digest protein for its calories—four per gram. While protein can be sacrificed for energy, it's not desirable. By using protein for calories, your body diverts it from its other responsibilities. Eating a well-balanced diet that includes adequate protein prevents this from happening. Inadequate protein, on the other hand, spurs your body to dismantle its own protein-packed tissues, including muscles and organs, in the hunt for amino acids to build body proteins. Even a small protein shortfall in your diet that persists for days spurs your body to turn on itself, decimating your lean tissue. A prolonged protein deficiency weakens your organ function, sapping your zest for life.

Studies show that protein intake begins to decline after age 50, and people over 70 eat the least amount of protein. Far too many seniors give protein-packed foods the heave-ho, often in hope of preserving heart health, since many foods rich in protein are packed with fat and cholesterol, too. But a multitude of foods contain the protein you need with just a trace of fat, including beans, most seafood, and nonfat dairy products, such as milk and yogurt.

The recommended dietary allowance (RDA) for protein is 56 grams (g) for males age 51 and older and 46 g for women in that age group. However, quotas are based on ideal body weight. That's why it may be more accurate to figure your own personal protein needs. Here's how: Multiply your ideal body weight by .36 to get the number of protein grams you should eat per day.

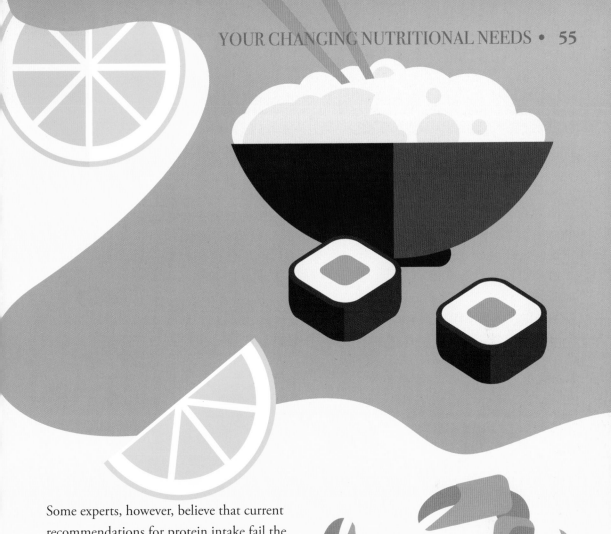

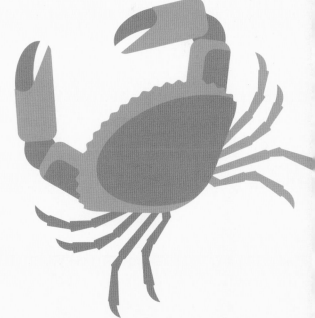

Some experts, however, believe that current recommendations for protein intake fail the over-50 crowd, especially those pushing 70 or more. Why? Because of the way you process protein as you get older. Your body is simply not as efficient as it was, and experts say that older people should probably eat more protein than the RDA suggests. Older adults lose protein stores with age and don't metabolize protein as efficiently. A better estimate of protein needs may be to multiply your ideal body weight by 0.45. This will provide you with the number of protein grams you must eat every day to impede the effects of age on your body. That's especially true if you're very physically active (that is, you do at least one hour of intense aerobic activity daily), as you may need even more protein to preserve muscle mass.

Getting enough protein every day helps prevent the loss of lean muscle tissue, which lowers your calorie-burning rate and saps your strength as you get on in years. Protein also boosts your immunity, so you may not get sick as often. When you lose muscle mass, it's difficult to regain it: While physical activity, particularly weight training, helps preserve the muscle tissue you have, it won't increase the size of your muscles that much.

But be careful with protein. People with liver and kidney disease, and those trying to manage diabetes, need the expert instruction of a registered dietitian to figure their protein needs. Too much protein is a drag on your system, taxing your organs, and even contributes to weight gain when you exceed your calorie needs.

FLUID

You need it, but your body can't make it in the amounts necessary to sustain life. That makes water absolutely essential, even though it's often shortchanged as a nutrient. You could go for days, even weeks, without food. That long without fluid would spell certain disaster.

If you weigh about 154 pounds, your body loses more than 10 cups of fluid a day—more if it's warm out or if you're exercising. Where does it all go? About half your body water is lost from your lungs and skin (you sweat all the time to maintain your internal temperature, even if you don't feel like you do). You lose the rest in urine and stool.

If you're like most people, you take your body for granted, expecting it to always work right. But if you don't feed it enough fluid, all bets are off. Fluid in the body aids the digestion, absorption, and transport of nutrients; ferries waste products away from cells; makes urine to get rid of toxins from the blood; builds tissue; regulates internal body temperature, so that you're not too hot or too cold; cushions joints and organs; and maintains blood pressure and fluid balance.

Health experts say that older people are prone to nutritional shortcomings that harm their health, and getting too little fluid is one of them. Hot weather and living at high altitudes both push fluid needs even higher.

Age blunts your ability to detect thirst. For that reason, older people must make a concerted effort to drink more fluids, even when not thirsty, to dodge dehydration. In addition, age diminishes your kidney's ability to retain water for your body to use, making you vulnerable to dehydration. In its milder form, dehydration can cause confusion, fatigue, headaches, weakness, flushed skin, and light-headedness, symptoms that may be so commonplace that you don't realize fluid loss is the cause. At its worst, dehydration results in dangerously low blood pressure (since blood is mostly water) and reduced kidney function that could spell disaster, especially if you are taking medications whose by-products must be eliminated through the urine. What's more, getting back on track after a bout of dehydration can take up to 24 hours, depending on how much fluid needs to be replaced.

Too little fluid is also linked to chronic conditions, increasing the risk for certain cancers, including those of the colon, breast, and urinary tract. Not getting enough fluid contributes to constipation, too. And inadequate fluid intake also increases the risk of kidney stones in people who are prone to them, including seniors. In fact, research suggests that people at risk for forming kidney stones, such as those who've had one in the past, should drink eight ounces of fluid with every meal, between meals, before bedtime, and when they get up at night to urinate. Researchers say this pattern of consistent fluid intake can prevent the reccurrence of kidney stones.

True, water is absorbed faster than any other fluid and put to use quicker in the body. But you may find drinking water a bit boring. Don't despair. Water isn't the only way to satisfy fluid needs. The recommendation for fluids includes water, seltzer, club soda, milk, juice, and herbal teas. Even coffee and regular tea can count toward satisfying fluid needs. (Although tea and coffee contain caffeine, a diuretic, more recent research shows that

they contribute to water balance in the body.) In addition, many foods are full of fluid, which counts toward dodging dehydration. For example, fruits and vegetables are up to 95 percent water by weight, so eating the recommended minimum of five servings a day helps keep you hydrated. Even pudding, gelatin desserts, ices, popsicles, frozen juice bars, ice cream, frozen yogurt, and sherbet may be counted as fluid because they are liquid at room temperature.

DECREASING NEEDS

There are only a few nutrients for which your needs decrease as you get older. But it's just as important to adjust your diet for these decreasing needs as it is for your increasing needs. Too much of these nutrients can be just as harmful to your health as too little of those in the previous section.

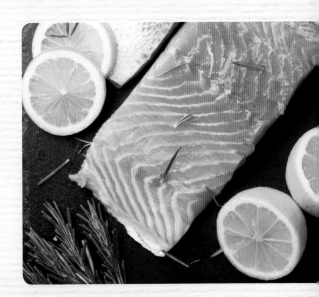

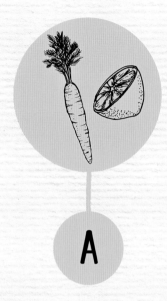

VITAMIN A

Vitamin A is everywhere in the body, despite the widespread perception that it's only good for vision. Ensuring immunity and keeping all tissues in top form are among its loftier functions. And, of course, vitamin A is vital for good vision.

Vitamin A comes in two varieties: retinol and carotenoids. Retinol is the ready-to-use form of the vitamin found in animal foods, including liver, eggs, and milk (due to vitamin A fortification). Carotenoids are plant-based raw materials that the body converts to active vitamin A. Beta-carotene is just one of the 50 or so carotenoids—found in plant foods including deep orange, yellow, and dark green fruits and vegetables—that the body can use to make vitamin A.

While the RDA of Vitamin A remains the same (3,000 IU for men and 2,300 for women), your ability to store vitamin A actually improves as you get older. Older people have higher levels of vitamin A on reserve in the liver, which is the reservoir for about 90 percent of all the vitamin A you have in your body, and they metabolize it at a slower rate. And older people have a higher concentration of vitamin A in the bloodstream when compared to younger people. As a result, older adults are more susceptible to vitamin A toxicity than younger adults.

Getting too much vitamin A hurts bone health. Just doubling the recommended vitamin A amounts increases your risk of hip fracture, which rises with age anyway due to osteoporosis.

Too much vitamin A also is toxic for your liver tissue. You'd probably need to take at least 25,000 IU of supplemental vitamin A every day for long periods before you'd develop a toxicity, and that's difficult to manage from food alone. However, if you're a fan of liver or fish liver oils, such as cod liver oil, you could induce a vitamin A overload. The signs of too much vitamin A in the body include headache, vomiting, hair loss, bone abnormalities, liver damage, and dry mucous membranes.

Carotenoids are not known to be toxic although high doses of beta-carotene may cause problems for smokers. It seems that as you take more, you absorb less. However,

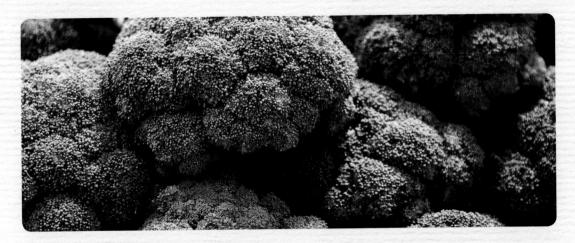

you may turn yellow or even orange with prolonged carotenoid consumption. When you reduce your intake of carotenoids, the color gradually disappears.

IRON

Iron is critical to the formation of healthy red blood cells. It's part of the red blood cell called hemoglobin, which is responsible for transporting oxygen to cells. And iron is part of myoglobin in the muscle, which can store oxygen until needed. Oxygen is key to energy production in the cells. Iron also bolsters the immune system, helps convert beta-carotene found in plant foods to vitamin A in the body, and participates in the production of amino acids, the building blocks of body proteins.

Despite iron's importance to health, if you are a woman, your need for it decreases as you age because iron stores in the body progressively increase. The recommended daily intake for adult men is 8 milligrams (mg). For women,

the RDA changes from 18 milligrams for women 19 to 50 to only 8 milligrams from age 51 on. Women who are still menstruating need more iron daily because nearly every bit of iron that's lost from the body is a result of bleeding. If you're taking hormone replacement therapy, ask your doctor about your iron status, since you may still have some blood loss.

Women who have struggled with iron-deficiency anemia all their lives—a disease caused by deficient iron stores—may find it odd that some people have too much iron on board. But the tables turn with age. If you're age 70 or older, you may be getting too much iron via fortified foods and supplements.

Iron overload means mayhem for your body. Excessive iron facilitates free radical damage to your cells, allowing these pesky forms of oxygen to convert low density lipoprotein (LDL, the "bad" cholesterol) into a variety that sticks to artery walls, plugging them up and restricting the flow of blood.

There are two forms of iron in foods: heme, present primarily in animal products; and nonheme, found mostly in plant foods. Heme iron is best absorbed by the body, so if you need more iron because you are still menstruating, make sure to include animal products in your diet and don't overlook fortified foods, including breads and cereals, as viable iron sources. Consuming plant-based foods fortified with iron along with vitamin C—found in foods such as orange juice, grapefruit, and tomatoes—enhances iron uptake by the body. If you still need extra iron, avoid drinking coffee and tea with meals, as they limit iron absorption.

CARRY ON WITH CAROTENOIDS

Just because you don't need more vitamin A with age doesn't mean you should avoid carotenoid-rich foods, such as carrots, cantaloupe, sweet potatoes, broccoli, and spinach. On the contrary. The body makes vitamin A from carotenoids on an as-needed basis, so the risk of overdosing on carotenoids from food is just about nil. That's in contrast to taking vitamin A supplements, which contain preformed vitamin A, called retinol. Too much retinol stored in the liver can be toxic.

Beta-carotene is one of 50 carotenoids that the body uses to prevent cataracts, head off heart disease, and curtail cancer, all of which become increasingly frequent with age.

Beta-carotene probably works as an antioxidant, fending off cellular damage that can mimic the effects of aging, slowing you down in your prime. How does a simple vitamin act as superhero? Beta-carotene probably traps and squelches free radicals, those destructive forms of oxygen that your body makes all day and all night as part of its metabolism. It may sound natural to produce free radicals, but it's not at all beneficial. Free radicals wreak havoc on cells' structure and genetic material, diminishing tissue and organ strength.

Supplementation with high doses of beta-carotene (more than 25 milligrams a day) is associated with adverse outcomes in heavy smokers.

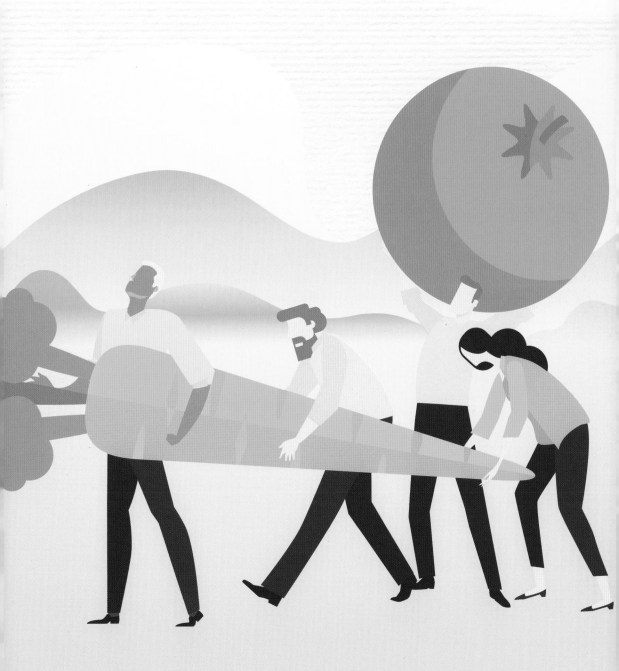

SODIUM

Sodium is often cast as the bad guy, but it plays an important role in your body. Sodium fosters fluid balance, makes sure muscles contract properly, and helps ferry nutrients into and waste products away from cells for excretion from the body.

But your body requires only minuscule amounts of sodium. Just 500 milligrams (mg) a day, the amount found in about one-fifth teaspoon of salt, is all it takes to keep your body running in top form.

To eat that little sodium is nearly impossible, however. That's because sodium is unavoidable; it's in nearly every food. Processed foods contain much more sodium than natural foods, however. In fact, an estimated 75 percent of all the sodium found in the American diet comes from highly processed foods, including canned soups, fast foods, snack chips, and frozen pizza. Because it's so hard to avoid sodium, an intake of 2,000 mg of sodium a day is not considered unhealthy for adults.

If you're trying to control high blood pressure, a concern for many older adults, then curb your sodium intake. A sodium-packed diet may aggravate high blood pressure and work against the medications you have been prescribed to control it. And a high-sodium diet often lacks potassium, a mineral that helps keep blood pressure in check.

Should you eat less sodium if you don't suffer from high blood pressure? That's debatable, but worthy of discussion. It's tough to say whether a low-sodium diet will decrease high blood pressure risk. We do know that a certain portion of the population, perhaps 10 percent or so, is sensitive to sodium. That means that a high-sodium diet boosts their high blood pressure more readily. And it's nearly impossible to tell who is sodium sensitive, since widespread testing of the general population is not feasible at this time. You also need to consider the fact that nearly everyone's blood pressure goes up somewhat with a high-sodium diet, perhaps to a level that is symptom-free yet dangerous to your health. (High blood pressure boosts your risk of heart attack and stroke.) Finally, a sodium-packed diet is rarely a well-balanced one overall, and it most likely leaves out the other myriad nutrients, including calcium, potassium, and magnesium, that researchers say conspire to keep blood pressure in line.

The CDC's 2015–2020 set of guidelines recommended that people do not exceed 2,300 milligrams (mg) of sodium per day—and they note that on average, Americans ingest 3,400 mg per day.

CALORIES

Calories are the energy in food that your body harnesses to fuel its own functions. During digestion, the body transforms food energy into glucose, the fuel that cells run on. Only three nutrients provide energy: carbohydrate, protein, and fat. Alcohol contains calories, too, but is not considered nutritionally necessary. Water, vitamins, and minerals are calorie-free.

Calorie needs are based on growth, body composition, and physical activity. As a baby, you required nearly four times the calories per pound as a 51-year-old. During adolescence, another period of tremendous growth, and throughout young adulthood, calorie needs increase dramatically to fuel the manufacture of millions of cells, build bone tissue, and make lean tissue, including muscles.

Needless to say, your calorie needs are lower after age 50, partially due to reduced physical activity, but mostly because of changes in body composition. As you age, lean tissue (mostly muscle) wanes. For example, muscle mass accounts for about 45 percent of total body weight during most of your adult life but declines to around 27 percent by age 70. And you may more than double your amount of body fat between the ages of 25 and 75.

What bearing do these body changes have on calorie needs?

Lean muscle mass burns more calories than fat. Muscle is a high-maintenance tissue, while fat is rather inert, not taking much energy for upkeep at all. So, if you have less muscle, which we all do with time, you need fewer calories to maintain your weight if your physical activity remains constant.

IN SEARCH OF FLAVOR

If you find yourself reaching for the salt shaker more often, it's probably not the fault of your cooking. You may need more salt to enhance the way food tastes because of your age.

As you get older, your ability to savor foods wanes. It's not your sense of taste so much as your sense of smell, which is largely responsible for flavor perception. Head injury, upper respiratory infections, and certain medications can also dull taste perception. (For more on sense of taste, see pages 29–30.)

Whatever the case, a blunted ability to taste foods may mean using more salt in search of flavor. The net result is too much sodium in the diet. If this scenario applies to you, a doctor's checkup may be in order.

Assuming light to moderate activity, men need 2,300 calories a day after age 50 (down from 2,900 daily before age 50); women 50 and older need 1,900 calories a day (down from 2,300 calories daily before age 50).

If you don't decrease your calorie intake or increase physical activity, you can easily pack on the pounds with time. Consider this: Just 100 calories a day more than you need to maintain your weight—about the amount in two ounces of chicken or a tablespoon of peanut butter—can pack on more than 10 pounds per year if you don't increase the amount of exercise you do.

Your mission: Do more with less. That means make calories count by choosing the most nutrient-packed, lowest-calorie foods you can most of the time. Don't worry, you're allowed some treats! Just choose them wisely.

To get the most from foods, choose whole grains and fortified cereals; take whole fruits over juices; delve into deeply colored choices, such as dark green, yellow, and orange vegetables, especially those from the cruciferous group such as broccoli, cauliflower, kale, and cabbage; eat at least three servings of low-fat dairy products daily; prepare a minimum of two bean meals instead of meat as a main dish twice weekly; and favor fish.

It's important to keep in mind that the daily calorie intake for people over 50 recommended by the Food and Nutrition Board of the National Academy of Sciences is merely a guideline, which is based on a woman who weighs 143 pounds and is 5 feet 3 inches tall and a male who weighs 170 pounds and is 5 feet 8 inches tall. You may need more calories, or fewer, to achieve and maintain a healthy weight. Ask your doctor for guidance about your weight.

Figure your own personal energy needs with the following calculation, which assumes that you get light to moderate activity every day:

- **FOR MEN:** Multiply your ideal weight by 13.5 to get daily calorie needs.

- **FOR WOMEN:** Multiply your ideal body weight by 13.2 to get daily calorie needs.

EXAMPLES:

A woman who weighs 150 pounds, but should weigh 140 to help head off diabetes and heart disease would need

150 pounds x 13.2 = 1,980 calories a day to maintain her weight

140 pounds x 13.2 = 1,848 calories to help lose weight gradually and safely

A man who has recently been ill and weighs 140 pounds, but who should weigh 170 pounds would need:

140 pounds x 13.5 = 1,890 calories daily to maintain his weight

170 pounds x 13.5 = 2,295 calories daily to gain weight gradually

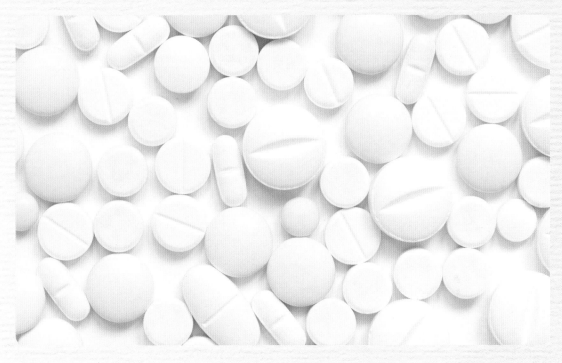

THE ROLE OF MEDICATION

If you're over age 50, you're most likely taking more medicine than you did when you were younger. That's because age increases the likelihood that you'll need to manage at least one chronic illness, including arthritis, diabetes, high blood pressure, and heart disease.

Not only do you raid the medicine chest more often as you age, you may take several different types of prescription and nonprescription drugs every day. Commonly used over-the-counter medications include aspirin, antacids, acetaminophen, ibuprofen, naproxen sodium, various cold remedies, antihistamines, and laxatives. The most commonly used prescription medications in the over-50 crowd are those such as digitalis, diuretics, and blood pressure pills that are used to control cardiovascular conditions.

The lure of medications is powerful. Who doesn't want to pop a pill, sip a liquid, or apply a patch to help ease annoying or painful symptoms? We're bombarded with advertisements for drugs in both the print and broadcast media. And new remedies seem to pop up on pharmacy shelves daily. In fact, more and more prescription drugs are now available in over-the-counter forms. Today there are more than 600 over-the-counter medications available to consumers—including powerful antihistamines and antacids—that required a doctor's prescription 20 years ago.

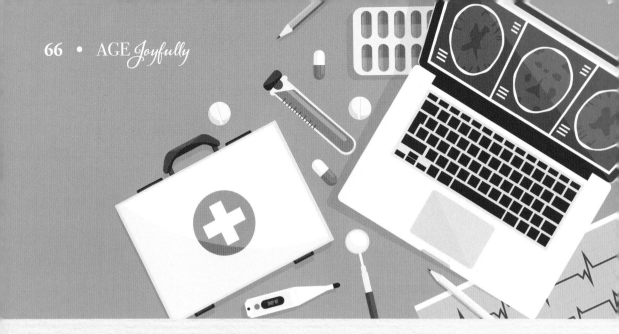

RISKS VERSUS BENEFITS

The increased availability and use of nonprescription medications, along with the increasing need for prescription medications as you age, has its downside, however. Combining medications increases the risk of drug-drug interactions that can have serious adverse effects. Some may be immediate and obvious; others may be insidious. For instance, many people give their body a double dose of potassium-leaching potions when they down diuretics and laxatives, whether they are prescription or over-the-counter medications. These two types of drugs both promote potassium loss, which can cause confusion and an irregular heartbeat. This may compound a preexisting potassium deficiency because of a diet low in fresh fruits and vegetables, whole grains, and dairy products.

It's generally better to employ a healthy lifestyle as a weapon against chronic illness, rather than to rely on pills to do it for us. For instance, losing weight can reverse the elevated blood glucose levels that are increasingly common with age, and it can help lower elevated blood pressure. And regular physical exercise can combat both conditions while actually helping to reduce arthritis pain by promoting flexibility and blood flow. Whenever possible, substitute a healthy habit for medication.

That said, it's not likely you'll be medication-free as time wears on. That's because no matter how healthy your lifestyle, increased longevity boosts the risk of chronic disease as well as minor aches, pains, and irritations. Given the multitude of drugs to prevent and treat chronic conditions, you and your doctor should carefully weigh the risks against the benefits of any drug. For example, when you've tried every lifestyle change in the book and your blood pressure or blood cholesterol remains high enough to harm your health, it's probably time to medicate. By the same token, perhaps getting a bit more rest, relaxation, and regular physical activity would help put the kibosh on minor tension headaches, which could reduce or eliminate your dependence on daily doses of aspirin or acetaminophen for pain relief.

It's important to be aware that every medication, no matter how benign you have been lead to believe, has side effects. Taking aspirin every day can result in blood loss from your gastrointestinal tract, inducing iron-deficiency anemia. Chronic aspirin consumption also leaches folate from your bloodstream. A folate deficiency stops cell replication, resulting in pernicious anemia while increasing your risk for heart disease. Daily doses of acetaminophen, often used to diminish the pain of arthritis, can cause blood loss and contribute to liver and kidney damage. Diuretics, used as therapy for high blood pressure, make it tough for your body to hang onto minerals, promoting excretion of potassium, magnesium, zinc, calcium, and chromium. Even the ubiquitous antacids you take to quell a queasy stomach push out phosphate. Phosphate loss leads to profound muscle weakness, pins and needles sensations, and even convulsions. And mineral oil, a common over-the-counter laxative, leads to losses of vitamins A, D, E, and K and the minerals calcium, phosphorus, and potassium from your body. The bottom line: Many medications can influence your health in other than their intended ways. Carefully contemplate every medication you use, and evaluate your arsenal of medications every so often with your doctor.

GET THE FACTS

Don't ignore the instructions your pharmacist provides with every prescription. Likewise, carefully read the fine print of the packages of over-the-counter drugs, no matter how familiar you are with them. They often change to reflect new findings about how to take a remedy. To best remember how and when to take your medication, request a written copy of instructions rather than relying on verbal communication for what you must do. (If you're like most people, you may forget once you leave the store, or as time wears on, you may need a refresher.) Always ask for help when you're confused. In addition, be sure to query the pharmacist about combining one or more prescription drugs and about taking nonprescription pills and potions along with prescription medications.

BODY CHANGES THAT INFLUENCE DRUG METABOLISM

As you age, body changes cause you to process medications differently. Getting older means the loss of fluid and lean tissue, including muscle, and an increase in body fat as a percentage of your total weight. These can all profoundly affect the way your body handles medications.

Your body composition is an important consideration in determining how you will respond to a drug. By the time you are 75 years old, you may have doubled the amount of body fat as a proportion of your body's makeup. Muscle mass accounts for nearly half of total body weight during most of your adult life but declines to about 25 percent by age 70. What's the significance of the changes? Many drugs are dissolved, transported, and stored in fat. When you have more fat in your body, you run the risk of accumulating fat-soluble drugs in your tissues. That means the drug hangs around longer than intended because it takes longer to be cleared from your system, increasing the risk for toxicity. By the same token, medications that require the watery compartments of your body for dissolution and distribution may also reach higher concentrations in the body, largely because there is less water to go around. Overall size matters, too. That's why a child would receive a much lower dosage of an antibiotic or pain killer than would a 40-year-old. Doctors take size into consideration when prescribing drugs.

The way your body handles drugs changes more and more as you get older. In addition to a decrease in body fluid and an increase in body fat, many age-related body changes discussed influence how you process and respond to drugs. For instance, getting older brings on a decrease in brain cells and a reduced blood flow to the brain, making you more susceptible to medications that can cause dizziness as a side effect, such as the glyburide often prescribed for type 2 diabetes control. This susceptibility can, in turn, result in falls and fractures. (Fractures are more likely with age because of osteoporosis.) Changes in hormone levels also make older people increasingly vulnerable to the side effects of certain medications, while a decline in lung elasticity may lead to a pronounced effect of other drugs. And a reduction in the strength of your immune system could mean you don't respond as well as you did previously to antibiotic therapy.

Older adults often need less of a drug to achieve effectiveness. In fact, if you're age 65 or older, the directions on over-the-counter drugs may not be appropriate for you. Designated dosages are often determined through scientific studies conducted with young and middle-aged adults, who have more lean muscle tissue mass and more water in their bodies. Ask your doctor about how much of any medication is right for you, and never take more than

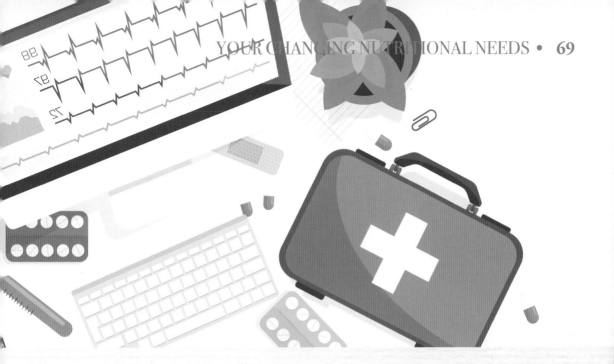

prescribed. As an aside, be sure to take the correct dose of a liquid medication by using a standard measuring spoon. Common tableware teaspoons can hold up to twice as much medication.

There's more. As you get older, there is a drop-off in albumin, a blood protein that helps maintain the body's fluid balance. This is important because lower albumin concentrations can affect drug metabolism. Drugs such as aspirin, the anticoagulant warfarin (coumadin), and the anticonvulsant phenytoin bind with albumin for distribution to body tissues via the bloodstream. Although a low-protein diet is one of the surest routes to low albumin levels in people of all ages, even the best diet doesn't protect older adults against decreased albumin levels. Low-protein diets in particular exacerbate a depressed albumin level and may mean even slower drug clearance from

the body. People with conditions that require carefully controlled protein intakes, such as kidney disease, must pay particular attention to their medications and the potential effect on their body.

One of the most vital organs for drug metabolism is the liver. As you get older, the liver becomes less efficient. It gets smaller and receives less blood. As a consequence, drugs stay in your body longer, leading to higher-than-desired concentrations of medications. After a while, excessive levels become toxic, decimating organs. For example, prolonged penicillin use in older people may mean higher blood levels of the drug, leading to kidney damage. In addition, some popular drugs for chronic conditions—such as gemfibrozil, which manages risk factors for heart disease—can actually damage the liver tissue. If you take these drugs, your doctor should conduct liver function tests (via a blood test) periodically to check for liver toxicity.

As you get older your kidneys get less blood, too, and they lose some of their ability to filter your blood for the toxic by-products of drug metabolism. Your kidneys have a harder time getting rid of drugs including atenolol, digoxin, gentamicin, methotrexate, penicillin, and tetracycline. A reduced kidney capacity is seen by some experts as the most important reason that older people process medications differently than their younger counterparts, although a combination of factors seems likely.

DODGING DRUG DOLDRUMS

You must be in tip-top nutritional shape to properly process medications and to avoid their nutritional side effects. This is especially true as you get older, as your body is less resilient and can withstand fewer of these effects, which have nothing to do with how they help manage acute and chronic illness.

Since many drugs affect nutrient needs, that makes it all the more important to get the nutrition you need every day. Studies show that older adults lack many nutrients, such as the B vitamins and the minerals calcium, zinc, and magnesium. Dietary deficits are often made worse by regular medication use. What's more, as you age you need additional amounts of some nutrients, including calcium and vitamin D, and it becomes absolutely

crucial that you make your quotas for others, such as vitamins B12 and folate, protein, and potassium, in order to stay in good health.

Drugs can affect the absorption of nutrients in the intestinal tract. Cholestyramine, which is used to lower elevated blood cholesterol levels, reduces the uptake of vitamins A, D, E, K, and folate as well as the carotenes, which help fight cell destruction and provide the raw material for vitamin A production in the body. Colchicine, an antigout therapy, inhibits vitamin B12 absorption, which can put you at risk for megaloblastic anemia and heart disease. And vitamin D deficiencies can be induced by drugs, including the sedative phenobarbital. Inadequate levels of vitamin D in the body reduce the absorption of calcium, jeopardizing bone health.

Medications can affect what—and how much—you eat, to the point of affecting your health. Steroids taken to reduce serious inflammation seen in autoimmune diseases and in conditions such as emphysema can stimulate your appetite to the point of significant weight gain. Others, including methotrexate, which is used to quash cancer and treat rheumatoid arthritis, and fluoxetine, which is used to treat depression, suppress the urge to eat—but sometimes just temporarily. Still others, including lithium carbonate, which is used to treat manic depression, result in a change in your sense of taste that often causes food aversions and may lead to weight loss. Antidepressants such as clonazepam and paroxetine can make your mouth dry or sore. If any medication you take is causing wild fluctuations in your weight, tell your doctor.

There may be other alternatives to these drugs that provide a remedy, minus the side effects.

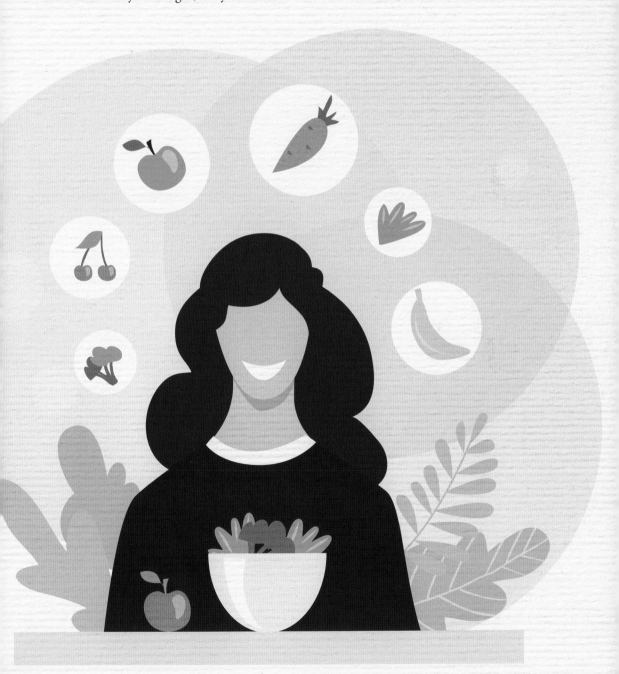

WHEN FOOD AND DRUGS DON'T MIX

It's hard to imagine a healthy food as a foe to your health, but when it comes to pharmaceuticals, there are some foods and medications that shouldn't be taken together.

Food influences how a drug is broken down and absorbed by your body, slowing it down or increasing its uptake. For example, taking acetaminophen for a headache or for arthritis pain right after a carbohydrate-rich meal significantly slows its absorption. Likewise, downing astemizole, an antihistamine, or the antibiotic azithromycin with food significantly limits their absorption from the intestinal tract. Drugs often compete with nutrients in the gut for absorption because they are ferried to the bloodstream by the same transport system. People who take levodopa and methyldopa to control Parkinson disease need to know that these drugs compete for absorption with the amino acids from protein digestion, which could result in the erratic effect of the drug.

Gulping grapefruit juice with your medications may not be so healthy after all. That's because grapefruit juice reduces the body's uptake of certain drugs, including vinblastine (a cancer therapy), losartan (for high blood pressure control), digoxin (for congestive heart failure treatment), and fexofenadine (to reduce allergy symptoms). Does that mean you should swear off grapefruit juice in the name of good health? No. Just wait a couple of hours after you take your pills to sip this vitamin C-filled beverage—or switch to orange juice, just to be on the safe side.

From a nutritional standpoint, you're encouraged to eat broccoli, cabbage, Brussels sprouts, and cauliflower because they are fat-free and packed with fiber, vitamins, and minerals. In addition, they contain indoles—plant substances thought to ward off chronic diseases, including cancer. So it's ironic that you may need to avoid these foods when taking certain medications. You see, indoles speed up drug metabolism. And so do the bioflavonoids found in citrus foods, which are best known for being rich in vitamin C.

Grilling foods over charcoal, which some claim is good for you because it's a low-fat cooking method, produces polycyclic aromatic hydrocarbons that also rev up drug metabolism in the liver. Ask your doctor or pharmacist about foods to avoid with your medications.

Alcohol is of particular concern. Chronic alcohol consumption results in deficiencies of the B vitamins, protein, magnesium, potassium, zinc, and vitamins C and D. Alcohol abuse weakens the immune system, and long-term use can lead to liver damage. And alcohol-drug interactions can be downright dangerous. Gulping alcohol and acetaminophen can be toxic to your liver tissue. Taking the medications that help lower blood sugar, such as glipizide, with alcohol can cause your blood sugar to plunge too low. And taking commonly prescribed anti-anxiety pills such as diazepam (Valium), lorazepam (Ativan), and alprazolam (Xanax) with an alcohol chaser can lead to excessive drowsiness, disorientation, and even death.

Even garden variety nonprescription antihistamines that quell cold and allergy symptoms make you much groggier when taken within a few hours of having an alcoholic beverage. In addition, when you have alcohol and medication in your system simultaneously, you are asking your liver to work overtime to break down and eliminate the by-products of both from your body. As you get older, this is not as easy for the liver to do and you may overtax it when you frequently combine alcohol and drugs.

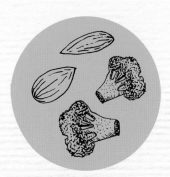

SUPPLEMENT SAVVY

Given the fact that many medications deplete your body of vital vitamins and minerals, taking extra as supplements is probably necessary to correct the effects of everyday drug use. There's little question that most people can take a multivitamin/multimineral preparation without any hazard to their health. The levels of nutrients in multis are usually kept to 100 percent of the daily value (DV), which presents little risk, even when you're taking most medications.

There are some drug-nutrient interactions that are so clear-cut, that whenever possible extra supplements should be started along with the medication to head off nutrient losses. Daily doses of the steroid prednisone to reduce inflammation necessitate getting extra calcium in your diet and in supplement form. That's because prednisone begins leaching calcium from your bones as early as eight days into the therapy, which may go on for months or years, depending on your condition. Simply taking an aspirin daily (on your doctor's advice) to ward off heart disease and stroke may render you low in the B vitamin folate, vitamin C, and iron (if the aspirin has resulted in small intestinal bleeds, which may go unnoticed), making a multivitamin necessary to pick up any slack in your diet.

Yet, while it seems intuitive, mixing vitamin and mineral supplements with one or more medications can be tricky. For instance, those who take digitalis to regulate their heartbeat should realize that large doses of supplemental vitamin D could work against the drug. Combining large doses of vitamin E (more than 400 international units a day) with aspirin and/or prescription anticoagulants is a prescription for disaster: All three work to thin

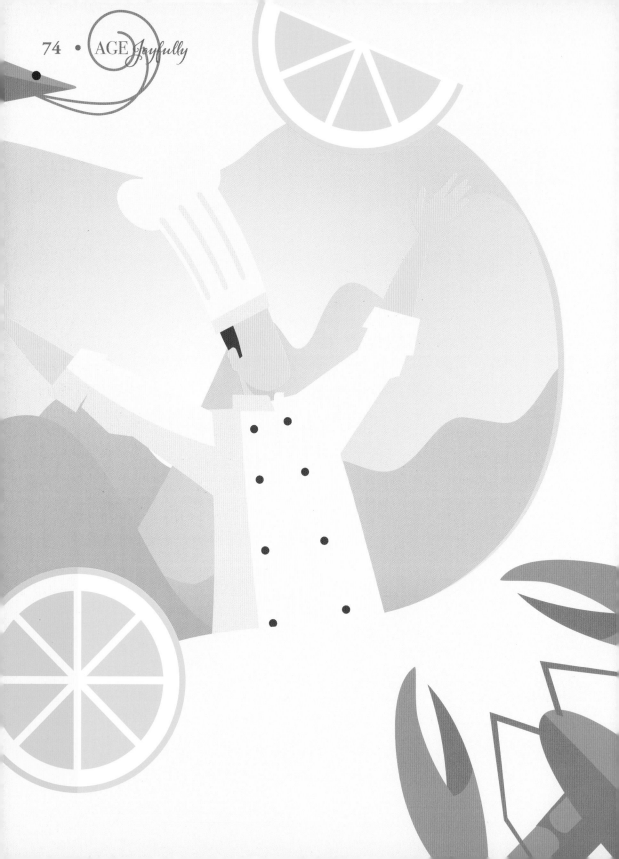

the blood, which may lead to uncontrollable bleeding. Consult a registered dietitian, a pharmacist, and your doctor to figure out what type of supplementation is right for you, given your medical history, current health, diet, and medications—both prescription and over-the-counter.

Combining herbs and drugs can be equally detrimental, although finding information about potential interactions is harder than scouting information about vitamins and minerals and medications. Part of the reason is the plethora of potential interactions between herbal preparations and other medications. Another reason is that people do not regard the herbs they take to help themselves relax, including kava kava and valerian, or to improve their memory, such as ginkgo biloba, as the medications that they are.

Herbal preparations are regulated as dietary supplements in this country. That means they do not have to prove their efficacy or safety, according to the Food and Drug Administration. By contrast, prescription and over-the-counter medications must go through a rigorous approval process. That lax attitude toward herbals provides a false sense of security, as consumers may see herbal preparations as harmless and not at all druglike. But nothing could be farther from the truth, especially since people purchase herbals in place of prescription and over-the-counter drugs. That can be a good thing, when properly researched. It may be much less costly and more convenient to

munch on candied ginger for a queasy stomach or motion sickness than to purchase a pill or a patch to ease those symptoms. And why not quaff some Echinacea for a few days when you feel a cold coming on instead of a costly antihistamine that may make you groggy? It's probably okay to opt for prophylactic feverfew pills to manage chronic migraines instead of relying on high-priced injections of antimigraine medication that may leave you with side effects.

Whatever their promise, you can't ignore the potential for harmful interactions between herbs and everyday medications you consume. For instance, if you take St. John's wort to deal with depression along with the prescription medication furosemide (Lasix), a diuretic to control high blood pressure, you can exacerbate the potassium depletion that furosemide causes. A potassium deficit jeopardizes your health, since it often results in confusion, weakness, and an irregular heartbeat.

Just because a pill or potion is derived from a plant doesn't mean it's free of side effects, nor does it make it automatically safe to consume with prescription and over-the-counter medications. And don't forget that the vitamins and minerals you take can potentially have detrimental effects on your body when all are taken together. Always consult your doctor about all of the pills, herbs, and vitamin and mineral supplements you take so that he or she has a complete picture.

A SUMMARY OF SOLUTIONS

Let's be honest: taking the time and attention to examine nutritional labels can be difficult. Here are some more general rules for staying healthy with food.

Eat a variety of foods to get a variety of needed vitamins and minerals. Focus on natural, whole foods rather than processed foods. Eat vegetables of different colors. Make your protein intake a mix of seafood (especially fatty fish), legumes, poultry, and lean red meat.

Include green, leafy vegetables and cruciferous vegetables in your diet on a regular basis. These foods are nutritional powerhouses. So are legumes, nuts, and seeds.

Talk to your doctor about food interactions if you are taking medications or supplements.

Consider a multivitamin. Consider taking a multivitamin to correct any deficiencies. Talk to your doctor first.

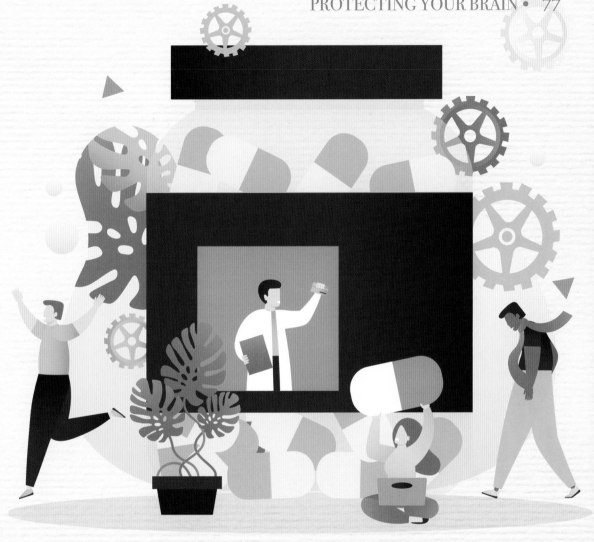

PROTECTING YOUR BRAIN

Many people worry about their mental acuity and memory as they age. In this chapter, we'll discuss how the brain works and how you can protect it physically, before the next chapter explores specific memory tricks you can learn to help your memory along.

HOW THE BRAIN WORKS

Every experience we have as we go about our daily lives creates a relay of signals across specific neurons and synapses in the brain. By experiencing something repeatedly—saying a name or phone number, seeing a face, practicing a golf swing, or making a recipe over and over again—we learn it. But how does the brain commit something to memory? When we experience something, a specific pattern of nerve cells, synapses, and neurotransmitters are activated. With each repetition, the participating cells and synapses actually begin to change and become better at relaying the signal. The neurons along the route may even sprout additional dendrites to create more and stronger synaptic connections. And in time the pattern becomes encoded in the brain as a long-term memory trace, like a well-worn path through the forest of neurons in the brain.

Research has begun to shed light on the types of physical changes that occur in the brain as a result of learning. For example, experiencing and learning lots of new things may increase:

- The development of new nerve cells in a region of the temporal lobe called the hippocampus, which is involved in learning and memory.

- The number and size of synapses—the connections between nerve cells that are necessary for relaying, processing, and recalling information.

- The amount of myelin insulation protecting the axons of nerve cells, especially in the bundle of nerves that allows the right and left sides of the brain to communicate.

- The number of tiny blood vessels that supply certain areas of the brain. More of these vessels means more blood and oxygen can flow to these areas to nourish nerve cells.

- The size and number of the glial cells that help to nourish and maintain the neurons in the brain and spinal cord.

These changes, taken together, highlight a very important feature of the brain known as plasticity. Plasticity refers to the way the brain is able to change as a result of experience. And it means that by exposing ourselves to new things and actively seeking more varied experiences on an ongoing basis, we can maintain and even enhance the brain's mental resources and cognitive abilities.

THE AGING BRAIN

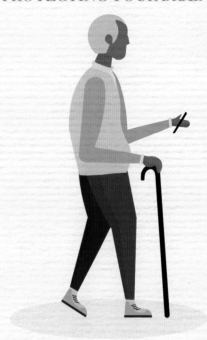

Time does appear to take a toll on the brain. Once we reach our 50s and 60s, our brains slowly lose mass, especially in areas such as the frontal lobes and hippocampus. The wrinkly cerebral cortex starts to get a little thinner. The number of synapses, or connections between neurons, tends to decrease. The brain pumps out less of the neurotransmitter chemicals that ferry signals across the synapses. And the number of receptors for those chemicals appears to decrease. Still, while we lose some brain cells here and there, especially in the deeper parts of the brain, we don't typically experience significant or widespread neuron loss unless a brain disease, such as Alzheimer's, is present.

In terms of cognitive functions, increasing age tends to make us a bit slower at processing information, learning new things, and retrieving information we've already stored, although once we commit something to long-term memory, it usually stays there just as well as when we were younger. We may struggle a bit more with remembering plans we made recently. And as early as our late 20s, our ability to recall the odd fact, name, or number starts a slow roll downhill. We may also become less adept at multitasking—trying to keep track of or work on more than one thing at a time—or switching quickly from one cognitive task to another.

Still, these gradual changes in cognitive function are not inevitable. Not everyone experiences them to the same extent—or even at all. Our brains and our cognitive abilities develop based on what we experience minute by minute, day by day, throughout our lives. And since no two people have exactly the same experiences (not even twins), no two brains are alike. Likewise, no two brains age—physically or functionally—in exactly the same way or at the same speed.

If you randomly invited a couple dozen healthy 70-year-olds into a room and tested their memory, problem-solving, and other cognitive abilities, you'd likely find considerable variation in the results. Most would have lost some degree of the mental sharpness they had when they were in their 20s. But some—perhaps four or five—would have barely lost a step and would perform as well or nearly as well as they did when they were in their 20s and 30s.

The point is that the brain's chronological age—the number of years it's been on the planet—is not necessarily the same as its functional age. While genetics no doubt plays a role in such variation, scientists believe that our differing experiences and choices—not just when we're young but throughout our lives—are major factors in how well our brains age.

And that's great news, because it means that even if you're no spring chicken, you can still make choices and take steps that will revitalize, challenge, and enrich your mind so that it can start working more like it used to.

ADDING ON

Scientists once thought that the brain could not create new neurons once it reached adulthood. And it's true that the brain does not have the regenerative ability of, say, the skin, which is constantly creating new skin cells and shedding dead ones and has considerable ability to repair and replace damaged areas. Damaged or dead nerve cells in the brain cannot be replaced. But recent research does indicate that the brain can grow new neurons in the hippocampus, an area that plays an important role in learning and creating new memories.

One of the most important ways you can help preserve and promote more youthful cognitive function throughout your life is to take good care of your brain's supply lines—the blood vessels that bring oxygen- and nutrient-rich blood to the billions of cells in your brain. That means shielding those vital supply lines by taking steps to prevent or control age-related diseases that can weaken or narrow them.

Your blood vessels are essentially tubes made of living tissue that are lined on the inside with a layer of tissue called the endothelium. The blood vessel walls start out strong and flexible, with endothelium that is smooth and unblemished, allowing blood to flow through freely and easily as the heart's contractions pump it around the body. As the years go by, however, a condition called atherosclerosis, or hardening of the arteries, can occur. Hardening of the arteries is a very common condition that often begins to develop before we even reach our teens and slowly progresses over time. Most often, it only begins to seriously threaten the brain, the heart, or other organs when we reach our 50s and 60s. Fortunately, you can beat back that threat by taking care of your brain and your body.

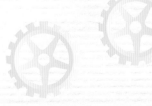

DIET

The best kind of diet for feeding your brain and maintaining healthy cognitive function is . . . drumroll please! . . . the same kind of diet that's good for your heart, your blood vessels, and the rest of your body. Despite what you may have read in a magazine or heard on some late-night infomercial, there are no miracle foods or magic diet plans that will suddenly send your IQ soaring or turn your memory into a steel trap. But that doesn't mean diet isn't important to brain health and cognitive function throughout your life. And it doesn't mean that there aren't foods and nutrients that may be especially helpful in protecting your brain cells and keeping them firing on all cylinders.

Think variety, balance, and moderation. These are the watchwords of a healthy diet for your brain. It, like the rest of your body, requires a plethora of nutrients to be healthy and to function well. So keep your food horizons wide. Plant-based foods, in particular, offer the body all sorts of phytonutrients—substances that appear to have protective effects on the body's tissues and organs. In general, the deeper or darker the color of the produce, the great its phytonutrient content. Fruits that falls in this category include berries, cherries, red grapes, raisins, plums, and prunes. Examples of deep-colored vegetables include broccoli, Brussels sprouts, kale, spinach, and beets.

Whole grains, beans, fresh fruits, and vegetables tends to be rich in nutrients, high in complex carbohydrates and fiber, and low in fat and cholesterol, so they deliver a lot of nutritional bang for your calorie buck. A diet in which these foods are center stage has been associated with a lower risk of stroke, heart and blood vessel disease, high blood cholesterol and triglycerides, high blood pressure, diabetes, and obesity—all conditions that can affect your brain along with the rest of your body.

RED AND BLUE

Research indicates that eating lots of blueberries and strawberries appears to slow cognitive decline in older folks, delaying it by as much as 2.5 years. Both fruits are loaded with phytonutrients called flavonoids that have anti-inflammatory and antioxidant powers. Getting more total flavonoids was also associated with a reduction in the degeneration of cognitive function that typically occurs when we get older.

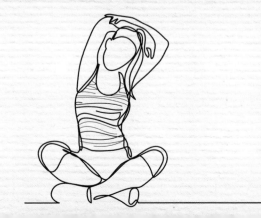

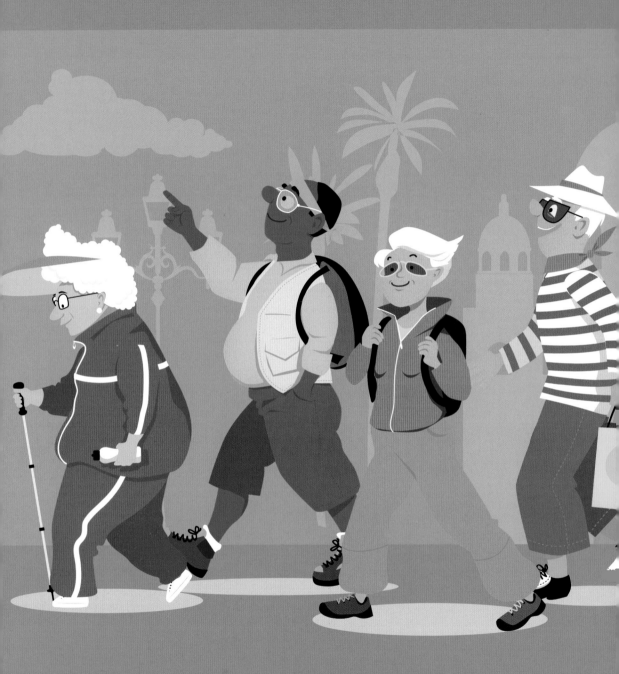

EXERCISE

Spending the day doing chores like mopping the floor, cycling to the post office, washing the windows, raking the leaves, and walking the dog may leave you rubbing your tired muscles and grumbling about feeling old, but it may be one of the most effective steps you can take to keep your brain from showing its age.

That's right. As surprising as it may seem, if you want to preserve good brain health and cognitive function as you grow older, you need to move your muscles. More precisely, you need to become more physically active every day and regularly engage in aerobic exercise—the kind that gets your heart and lungs working harder to meet your moving muscles' increased demands for oxygen.

As we discussed in chapter 1, exercise can help improve just about every aspect of your physical health, from boosting your cardiovascular fitness to lowering your risk of certain cancers. Experts have known for years that being more physically active lowers the risk of multiple medical issues that jeopardize the health of your brain, including obesity, diabetes, high blood pressure, low HDL cholesterol, hardening of the arteries, heart attack, and stroke. Regular exercise is also an essential part of controlling, treating, and/or recovering from these conditions. And now, based on a body of evidence that continues to expand, we know that being physically active can help lower the risk of Alzheimer's disease and other dementias and keep your mind sharp even into old age.

Some of the earliest research in this area, conducted in the 1990s on mice, showed that animals given time to run on a treadmill grew twice as many new neurons in the hippocampal region of their brains as did mice that didn't have access to treadmills. The hippocampus is a key player in learning and memory. When the researchers went back and taught both groups of mice how to navigate a maze, they found that the mice that exercised were quicker to learn and ended up taking a shorter path to the maze's end compared to the less active mice.

In another study, one group of middle-aged and older monkeys ran on a treadmill for an hour a day five days a week and another group simply sat on the machine for the same amount of time. In subsequent testing, the monkeys that exercised were twice as quick to learn new things as were the monkeys who were couch—or is that treadmill?—potatoes. The exercise benefit held true for even the oldest of the monkeys. The research further indicated that the active older monkeys only held on to their cognitive edge if they continued to exercise; with just a three-month break from exercise, the beneficial brain changes from activity disappeared.

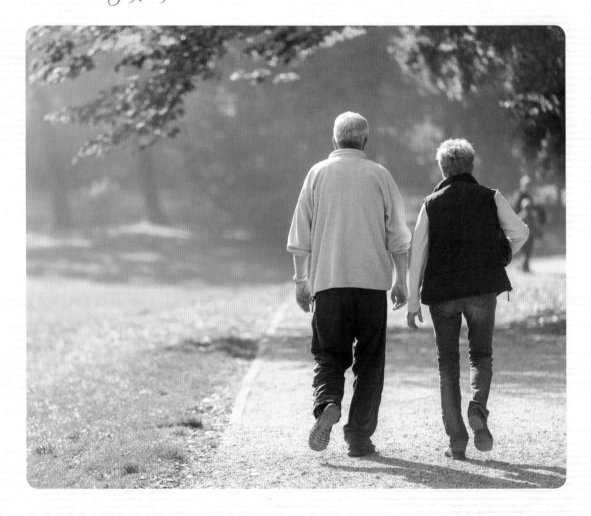

Research with people points to a very similar relationship between physical activity and cognition. Studies have found, for example, that people who exercise frequently have a distinctive brain-wave pattern characterized by steep peaks and valleys, which is associated with alertness. These active folks are better at focusing and blocking out distractions, which in turn means that they are better able to pay attention to information that they want to remember and better at retrieving those memories as needed.

Research has also found that aerobic exercise can help maintain short-term memory, especially verbal memory, which is important when you want to recall names, directions, and phone numbers, or match a name with a face. It also appears to greatly benefit functions such as planning, scheduling, and multitasking.

MAKE YOUR DAYS MORE ACTIVE

A simple way to start turning an inactive life into a more active one is to start small. Try some of these suggestions for including more physical movement into your days:

- Walk around your house, yard, or office while talking on the phone.

- When meeting up with friends, walk and chat instead of just sitting.

- Use stairs instead of elevators and escalators, especially when you're only going up or down a level or two. If you're going farther than that, get off a couple floors early and take the stairs the rest of the way.

- For nearby errands, leave the car in the garage and walk or take a bicycle.

- If you drive to work or to go shopping, choose the farthest parking spot from the building's entrance.

- At work, take a five-minute walk outside or even around the building itself instead of just sitting down during break times. Split your lunch hour and spend half eating your lunch and the other half taking a walk or climbing stairs.

- Instead of calling or emailing a coworker who sits in a different area of the building, walk over to them to ask a question or deliver information.

- Walk down every aisle of the grocery store, even if you only need a couple of things. (If you're worried about being tempted into buying sweets or snacks you don't need, just skip those specific aisles.)

- Take your dog for a walk two or even three times a day. If you don't own a dog, consider adopting one, volunteering as a dog walker at a shelter, or asking a neighbor if you can tag along as they walk theirs.

- Walk on a treadmill or just walk in place as you watch TV.

- Do your own housework (skip the robotic vacuum) and yard work. Consider using a push mower instead of one powered by electricity or gas.

- Wash your car the old-fashioned way—with a hose, a bucket, soap, and a sponge. Give yourself a real workout by waxing it by hand, too.

- Instead of going out to movies or shows, do something active like dancing, bowling, or playing miniature golf. Spend an hour or two strolling a museum, craft show, or flea market.

- Walk the grandkids around the zoo or a park, fly a kite with them, or join in their game of hide-and-seek.

◆ Take up an active hobby, such as bird-watching, metal detecting, woodworking, or gardening. Try recruiting friends for weekly games of bocce, horseshoes, or table tennis.

◆ Practice yoga, Pilates, tai chi, or some other form of relaxing movement. Virtually every health club, YMCA, and adult education program offers classes that teach such activities. Many hospitals do, as well.

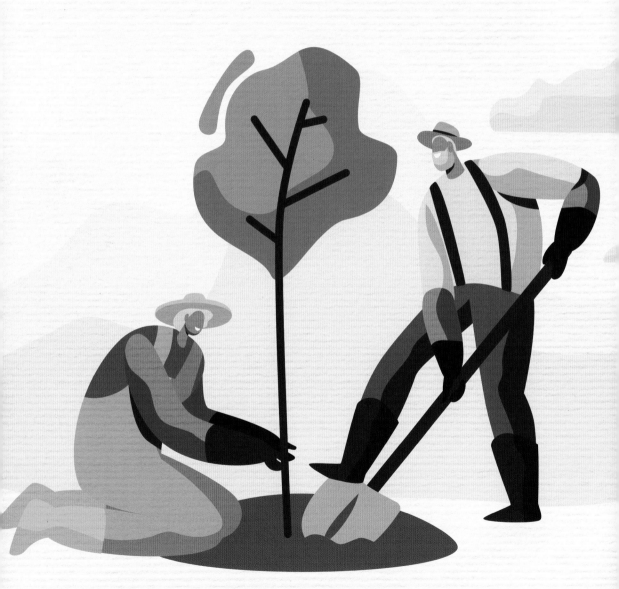

GET IN THE EXERCISE HABIT

Adding more movement to your days in such simple ways can certainly get you out of your easy chair and help you burn some extra calories. But it's not enough if you really want to revitalize and protect your brain. For that, you'll need to regularly engage in physical activities that are a bit more challenging. In other words, you'll need to exercise. And you'll need that exercise to be aerobic, meaning it works the large muscles of your arms, legs, and buttocks in repetitive movement and raises your heart and breathing rates for an extended period of time.

Aerobic exercise is the type that has shown so many positive health effects for your brain and blood vessels as well as your body as a whole. That's not to say that other forms of exercise, such as strength training or yoga, aren't beneficial. But to generate the kind of anti-aging changes for your brain that we've talked about in this chapter, you need to perform aerobic exercise several days a week. Researchers confirmed this when they studied two groups of sedentary (but otherwise healthy) adults aged 55 to 80. One group walked for 40 minutes three days a week for a year while the other engaged in strengthening and balance exercises for the same amount of time. The hippocampus region of the brain normally loses about 2 percent of its size each year as we age. When the researchers used

MRI to scan the brains of the two groups at the end of the study, they discovered that the hippocampus in folks who walked actually increased an average of 2 percent in size, while those who did the strengthening and balance activities lost 1 percent of their hippocampal volume. It's important to note two other findings that came out of this study. One is that an aerobic activity as simple and accessible as walking can help keep the brain young. The other is that even adults who only begin exercising regularly in their later years can reap its benefits for the brain.

GIVE IT A REST

Just as diet and exercise are important for your brain, so is sleep! Your brain never really stops working, even when you are asleep. As a matter of fact, when you're sleeping, it continues its job of keeping your basic body systems running smoothly.

This sleepy time cleanup routine is essential to alertness, concentration, learning, and memory during your waking hours. If you don't get enough quality sleep, your brain and cognitive functions suffer. Recent research in mice has found that lack of sleep can actually cause permanent damage to and even kill nerve cells in the brain, specifically a type that helps to keep us awake and aware. (The researchers believe similar damage occurs in the brains of humans who stay awake too long, too.)

So ensuring that you get enough high-quality sleep is not only important for your body, it's key to the health of your brain and your ability to think, learn, and remember.

YOU'VE GOT RHYTHMS

Before the invention of electricity, people went to bed shortly after the sun went down. Sure, it sounds boring, but there was a predictable rhythm to life that was dictated by sunshine and darkness. But in modern times, we tend to move to a different beat. Our frenetic lifestyles have disrupted the traditional rhythms of sleep. Sleep now competes against work and other commitments, along with a host of entertainment options. This creates challenges for us in terms of getting the rest we need.

Fortunately, we have a built-in body clock that attempts to keep us in step with a normal 24-hour cycle of waking and sleeping. This body clock is often referred to as the circadian rhythm. It is our body's natural way of trying to regulate not only our sleep patterns but a variety of other bodily processes, including digestion, elimination, growth, renewal of cells, and body temperature. When we work with our body's natural cycle, we can greatly improve not only our sleep but our overall health. When we fight against that cycle, on the other hand, our sleep, waking performance, and health can suffer.

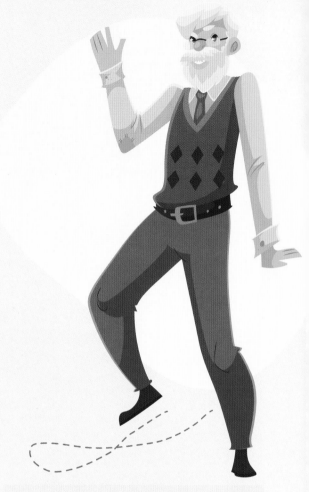

WHAT HAPPENS DURING SLEEP?

It was widely believed until about midway through the twentieth century that there was only one type of sleep. Whether you got one hour or ten hours of sleep, it was the same garden variety. And that is how most people still think of sleep today. But since the invention of modern machines that can monitor our sleep patterns, we have learned that there are actually two main kinds of sleep—an important discovery that has helped us gain insight into what happens during sleep.

One kind of sleep is called rapid-eye-movement (REM) sleep. It gets its name from the distinctive shifting of the eyes that occurs when you are in this state. The second kind is termed non-REM (NREM) sleep, during which the distinctive rapid eye movements are absent. NREM sleep is often very deep, involving both mental and physical inactivity. As you sleep, you cycle in and out of REM and NREM.

NREM sleep is further divided into four stages. You repeatedly pass through these stages for different lengths of time during a typical night's sleep. When you finally awaken, you have covered much ground without being aware of it. Had you been physically active all that time, you would be exhausted. But, interestingly, this very cycling through stages is what renews your body and mind while you sleep.

AGE AND SLEEP

Answer true or false about the following statement: Seniors don't need as much sleep as they did when they were younger. Most people would say "true." And most people would be wrong. It is a myth that seniors need less sleep simply because they are older. Older adults require the same six to nine hours of restful sleep as other adults. The stumbling blocks for seniors in getting this amount of sleep include poor lifestyle habits and chronic illness, both of which can disrupt sleep.

It used to be thought that the internal body clock of older people required them to get less sleep. Research has shown this notion to be false. It is true that seniors tend to rise earlier in the morning and become sleepy in the afternoon. This is due to the internal body clock setting itself to a different rhythm as we age. Social factors, such as going to bed early out of boredom, and medical illnesses and medications that cause fatigue and sleepiness, may also cause earlier bedtimes and therefore early morning awakening.

SET THE STAGE FOR BETTER SLEEP

In order to maximize your sleep time, there are four main considerations. You must:

- Begin your preparations for sleep during the day

- Schedule your sleep patterns deliberately

- Practice habits that help your body to relax before sleep

- Control your sleep environment

PREPARE FOR SLEEP ALL DAY

From the moment you wake up in the morning, you have choices to make that can affect how well you sleep that night. Making wise choices throughout the day can help you sleep soundly at night and awaken with renewed energy.

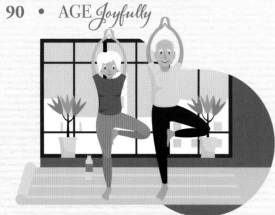

1. EXERCISE TO SLEEP BETTER

The majority of people claim that they don't exercise on a regular basis because they are too tired. Hmmm. Could that have something to do with sleep habits, perhaps? Chances are good that it does. If there were a competition to determine which lifestyle habit would win the title of "best intention never acted on," exercise would probably win. The reason we intend to exercise is that we all know how good it is for us. And research finds new benefits every day. Regular exercise improves heart health and blood pressure, builds bone and muscle, helps combat stress and muscle tension, and can even improve mood. Add one more benefit: sound sleep. Did you know that exercise can help you sleep sounder and longer? It's true. But the key is found in the type of exercise you choose and the time you participate in it during the day. What time of the day do you think exercise would best help you sleep? Morning? Afternoon? Evening? Right before bed?

Exercising vigorously right before bed or within about three hours of your bedtime can actually make it harder to fall asleep. This surprises many people; it's often thought that a good workout before bed helps you feel more tired. In actuality, vigorous exercise right before bed stimulates your heart, brain, and muscles—the opposite of what you want at bedtime. It also raises your body temperature right before bed, which, you'll soon discover, is not what you want.

Morning exercise can relieve stress and improve mood. These effects can indirectly improve sleep, no doubt. To get a more direct sleep-promoting benefit from morning exercise, however, you can couple it with exposure to outdoor light.

When it comes to having a direct effect on getting a good night's sleep, it's vigorous exercise in the late afternoon or early evening that appears most beneficial. That's because it raises your body temperature above normal a few hours before bed, allowing it to start falling just as you're getting ready for bed. This decrease in body temperature appears to be a trigger that helps ease you into sleep.

The type of vigorous workout we're talking about is a cardiovascular workout. That means you engage in some activity in which you keep your heart rate up and your muscles pumping continuously for at least 20 minutes. Although strength-training, stretching, yoga, and other methods of exercise are beneficial, none match the sleep-enhancing benefits of cardiovascular exercise

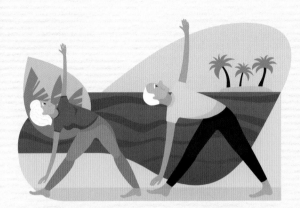

2. BRIGHTEN YOUR MORNING

Light tells the brain it is time to wake up. That's probably obvious to anyone who has had to turn on a light in the middle of the night and then has had trouble getting back to sleep. What may not be so obvious is that exposure to light at other times, particularly in the early morning, can actually help you sleep at night.

How does morning light improve sleep? The light helps to regulate your biological clock and keep it on track. This internal clock is located in the brain. There does, however, appear to be a kind of forward drift built into the brain. By staying up later and, more importantly, getting up later, you reinforce that drift, which means you may find you have trouble getting to sleep and waking up when you need to. To counter this forward drift, you need to reset your clock each day, so that it stays compatible with the earth's 24-hour daily rhythm—and with your daily schedule. Exposing yourself to light in the morning appears to accomplish this resetting.

Many factors can affect our biological clock, but light appears to be the most important. The timing of exposure is crucial; the body clock is most responsive to sunlight in the early morning, between 6:00 and 8:30 A.M. Exposure to sunlight later does not provide the same benefit. The type of light also matters, as does the length of exposure. Direct sunlight outdoors for at least one-half hour produces the most benefit. The indoor lighting in a typical home or office has little effect.

3. MANAGE STRESS

If you moved into a new neighborhood only to discover that it was plagued by smelly smoke from a nearby factory, you would likely be annoyed or angry at first. But after several weeks, you probably wouldn't notice it as much. You would become conditioned to the smell despite the fact that it may not be terribly healthy for you. A similar phenomenon can occur when we experience stress on an ongoing basis. We may be so bombarded with daily stress that we become accustomed to it. But such constant exposure to stress can

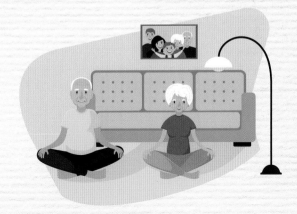

make it difficult to get needed sleep and can compromise our overall health.

It's important to dispel the myth that you can avoid stress. If you breathe, you are going to encounter life situations that bring stress. Since you can't avoid it, the best option is to learn to manage it. One key to managing stress is assessing what you have control over and what you don't. For instance, if your boss has set an unrealistic deadline for a project, you may have little or no control over changing that. But you do have control over how you respond to that deadline. And your response to a given situation is what you want to focus on as you seek to manage stress. You can choose to do certain things and not others. This ability to choose puts you in control and gives you the ability to make the situation work for you.

Professional therapists who specialize in stress reduction will tell you that your body is the best guide to determining when you are feeling stressed. If you pay attention to how you feel both physically and emotionally, you can often intervene before stress begins to interfere with your sleep.

What does stress management during the day have to do with sleeping well at night? Plenty. Have you ever had the unpleasant experience of crawling into bed exhausted and spending the next few hours tossing and turning as you go over every detail of your day? That is stress at work on your mind. All of those emotions

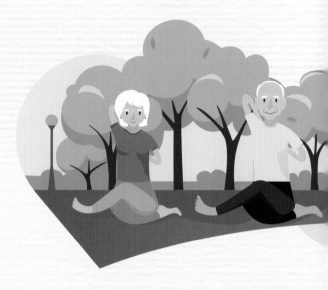

and thoughts throughout the day that were not dealt with at the time can work their way to the surface in the quiet of night.

In addition, the more you dwell on the upsetting events, the greater the effect on your body. When it senses stress, the brain sends a message to the body to release hormones that heighten alertness and prepare it for action. This is known as the fight-or-flight response. It's a beneficial reaction if you need to fight off a dog that threatens you on your walk or jump out of the way of a speeding vehicle. But when the stress is mental and there is no physical response necessary, that heightened state of alertness can keep you from relaxing enough to sleep. By learning to deal with stressors in your life more immediately during the day, you are less likely to be kept awake by them at night.

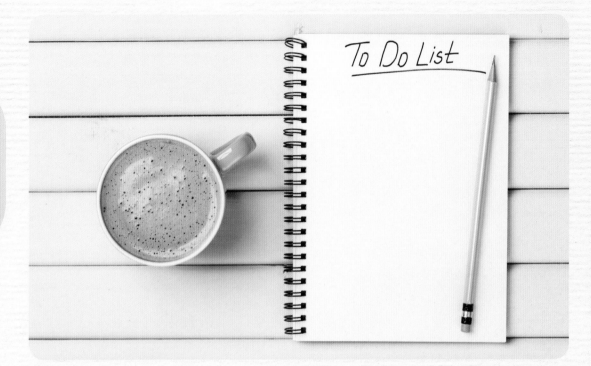

4. DON'T PROCRASTINATE

Many of us are great procrastinators, living by the motto "Why do today what I can put off until tomorrow?" If you're a procrastinator, you can't afford to put off reading this section. Putting work, projects, or tasks off almost always has bad consequences, one of which is disturbed sleep. Getting your work done can be seen as another way of managing your stress. You can choose to put your time and energy into accomplishing what is before you and reap the benefits or put it off and worry about it. Tasks left undone can even intrude into your dreams at night and, in extreme cases, lead to nightmares.

Avoiding procrastination takes some discipline. There are certain techniques, however, that can help:

◆ Make a "to do" list for the day. Then rank your list from most to least important. Start with the most important and work your way through. If unexpected circumstances limit what you can accomplish that day, you will have put your limited time and energy toward the most important tasks. And this will leave you with a sense of accomplishment.

◆ Keep promises to do tasks on time. Make schedules and stick with them. When promised work is late, it only becomes more difficult to face as time goes by.

◆ Finish what you start. Leaving projects half done is sometimes worse than not starting them at all. An incomplete job will occupy your mind and make relaxing difficult. Also, work that is partly done robs you of the satisfaction that comes with closure.

◆ Learn to say "no." Sometimes we procrastinate because we feel overwhelmed by all of our commitments. Still, we continue to volunteer for tasks or projects because we don't want to tell someone "no." To combat this habit, make an effort to look realistically at your schedule and responsibilities before you commit to optional activities, and realize that knowing when to say "no" is better for your sleep and your health than worrying about tasks you can't hope to accomplish.

5. NAP SPARINGLY

Some people swear by naps; others find that napping during the day disrupts their sleep at night. The urge to nap is greatest about eight hours after we awaken from a night's sleep. This is when our body temperature begins the first of two daily dips (the other, more dramatic dip, occurs at night). A short nap in the early to middle afternoon can bring a renewed sense of energy and alertness. A nap in the late afternoon or early evening, on the other hand, can disrupt your sleep cycle and make it difficult to fall asleep when you retire for the night.

To benefit most from a nap, take it no later than mid-afternoon and keep it under 30 minutes. If you nap for a longer period, your body lapses into a deeper phase of sleep, which can leave you feeling groggy when you awaken. If you are severely sleep-deprived and can't go on without a nap, it is better to sleep for a longer time to allow yourself to go through one complete sleep cycle. An average sleep cycle takes about 90 minutes in most people.

If you find you need a nap every day, take it at the same time so your body can develop a rhythm that incorporates the nap. It's also possible to use naps to temper the negative effects of an anticipated sleep deficit. For instance, if you know you are going to be up late because of special plans, take a prolonged nap of two to three hours earlier in the day. This has been shown to reduce fatigue at the normal bedtime and improve alertness, although it may throw off your normal sleep rhythm temporarily.

6. EAT AND DRINK WISELY

How much of a direct effect diet has on sleep is still unclear. It's safe to say, though, that a balanced, varied diet full of fresh fruits, vegetables, whole grains, and low-fat protein sources can help your body function optimally and help ward off chronic conditions such as heart disease. And since chronic diseases and the drugs required for them can interfere with sleep, eating wisely can help you safeguard your health and your sleep.

Adjusting your eating routine may also help you get a better night's sleep. Most people in this country eat a light breakfast, a moderate lunch, and a large meal in the evening. Yet leaving the largest meal to the end of the day may not be the best choice, since it can result in uncomfortable distention and possibly heartburn when you retire for the night. You might want to try reversing that pattern for a more sleep-friendly meal plan:

- Eat a substantial breakfast. Because you are breaking your nighttime fast and consuming the nutrients you will need for energy throughout the morning, breakfast should be your largest meal of the day. Whole-grain breads and cereals, yogurt, and fruit are just a few examples of good breakfast choices.

- Opt for a moderate lunch. Choose brown rice, pasta, or whole-grain bread and a serving of protein—fish, eggs, chicken, meat, or beans.

- Finish with a light dinner. It is particularly important to eat lightly for your evening meal in order to prepare for a good night's sleep. Plan to finish your meal at least two hours before going to bed, preferably longer.

In addition, you may want to try these tips:

- Reduce or eliminate caffeine, especially in the late afternoon and evening. Caffeine is a stimulant, which is why so many of us reach for that cup of coffee in the morning to get us going. And it's true that some individuals can drink caffeinated beverages all day long and still sleep soundly at night. But if you're having trouble sleeping, then limiting your caffeine intake should be one of the first steps you try to help improve your sleep. Be aware that coffee is not the only source of caffeine. Many sodas and teas, chocolate, and some medications, especially those for headaches, also contain caffeine. Check labels to help eliminate such sources of stimulation.

- Some people are sensitive to the flavor enhancer and preservative monosodium glutamate (MSG). In susceptible individuals, it can cause digestive upset, headaches, and other reactions that can interfere with sleep. MSG is found in some processed foods and in some Asian foods. Try avoiding foods that contain MSG to see if it helps you sleep better.

- Drink the majority of your fluids for the day by the end of dinner. A full bladder may be cutting into your sleep time. Drink plenty of water throughout the day. Water is essential to healthy bodily functions. Shoot for eight glasses, or two quarts, per day. But be sure to drink the majority of your fluids before dinnertime so you won't be making numerous trips to the bathroom during your sleeping hours. Skip the alcohol. Despite making you feel drowsy, alcohol may actually be disturbing your sleep.

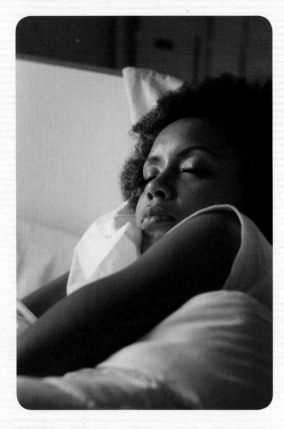

SCHEDULE YOUR SLEEP

It might seem unnatural to schedule your sleep like you would an important appointment, but this is one of the most vital principles to getting a good night's rest. Most of us begin our day with a morning routine. It helps us prepare ourselves physically and mentally for the day. So why not establish a bedtime routine that helps to prepare you for sleep? The purpose of a bedtime ritual is to send a signal to your body and mind that it's time to sleep. You probably already have some regular bedtime habits, even if you haven't realized it.

Brushing and flossing your teeth, lowering the thermostat, and setting your alarm clock may all be part of your evening routine. To help you get to sleep, you should perform these activities in the same manner and order every night. Establishing some type of bedtime ritual also provides closure to your day and allows you to go to bed and sleep with a more quiet body and mind.

Some people think going to bed on a schedule is only for children. While it's good for children to have a regular bedtime, it's also very good for adults who want to sleep like children when they hit the sack.

This regularity helps set your internal sleep-wake clock. Within weeks of keeping a regular sleep-wake schedule, you will begin to feel more alert than if you were keeping a variable sleep/wake routine. Not only will a stable rhythm of sleeping and waking improve the quality of your sleep, but it will probably also improve the quality of your life. Try it for six weeks to gauge the difference it makes in your energy and alertness.

EASE INTO SLEEP

Now that you know how to prepare for sleep during the day and schedule it at night, you're ready for bed. But before you peel those sheets back, consider how you might prepare your body and mind for that relaxing and peaceful sleep for which you long. The hour before bedtime is the most critical for good sleep.

When used properly, the time right before bed can help you let go of the stressful, anxiety-provoking events of the day. But if that last hour before slumber is not used properly, it can set the stage for a long night of tossing and turning. Try some of the following ideas to see which work best for you.

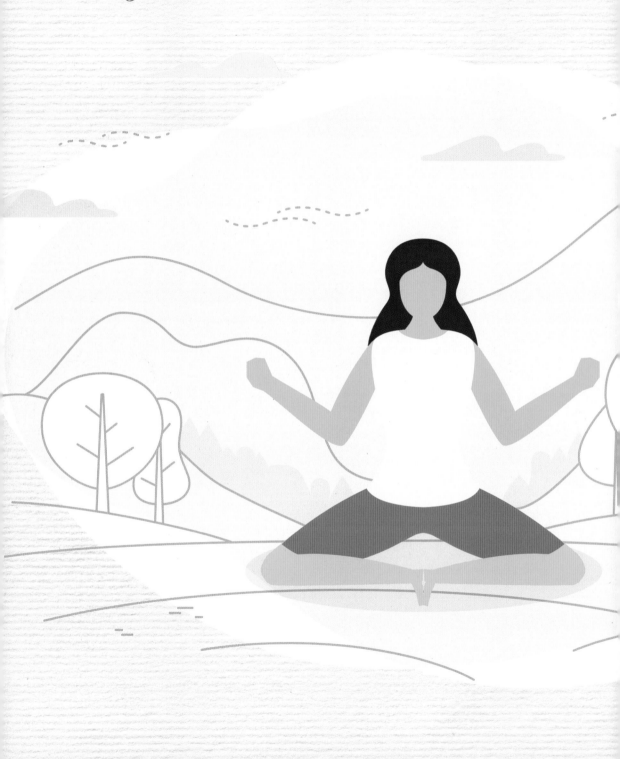

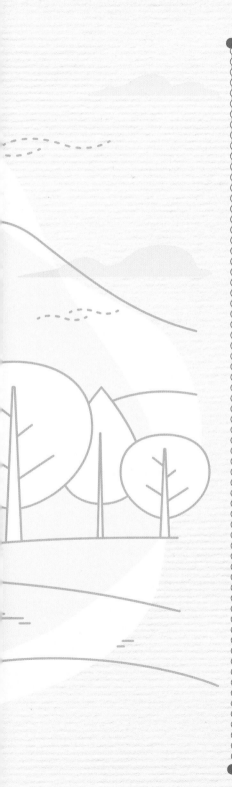

1. SEEK SERENITY

The key to preparing for sleep is to establish an atmosphere of peace and calm. Ease your mind and body with quiet yet pleasurable activities. You will create a sense of inner well-being that allows sleep to come quickly and easily.

- **Read to relax.** But choose your reading material with care. The idea is to read something light that won't stimulate your mind. In other words, you probably don't want to crack that new software manual. Better choices would be a popular magazine, a short story, or perhaps devotional reading.

- **Listen to music.** Choose music that relaxes you. In general, soft instrumental music has the most calming effect. Hard driving rock and pop beats often pull you into the music, causing you to be more awake, especially if the tunes are familiar. Another sound alternative might be playing a recording of nature sounds.

- **Try meditation or prayer.** These activities, which help many people relax, can also help you be at peace with whatever is on your mind.

- **Watch television,** but only if it helps you relax. Watching television is fine if you use some discipline. Falling asleep with the TV on is not the best way to start your sleep. In most cases, you have to awaken to turn it off, which forces you to have to fall asleep again. The idea is to stay asleep once you doze off. A better use of television is to watch it earlier in the evening and practice other relaxation techniques right before bed. If you must watch right before bed, don't watch in your bedroom.

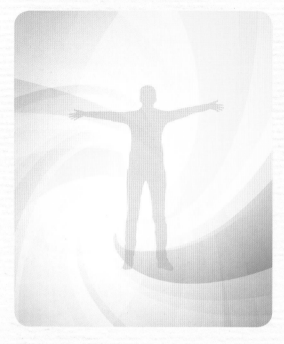

3. LET IT GO

You've just gotten off the phone with a relative who infuriates you every time you talk with them. Flying into your bedroom like a whirlwind, you try to get ready for bed. You lie down on the bed and repeatedly slam your fist into your pillow as you try to find a comfortable position. But you can't fall asleep. Too often people go to bed when their mind is a raging fury, agonizing over some event of the day. When your emotions are boiling over, stay out of the bed and the bedroom until you cool down. Try journaling or writing your frustrations down on paper to help unburden your mind.

2. TAKE A WARM BATH

One popular way to relax the body and slow down the mind is a warm bath, and you may find it fits the bill for you. But you may want to do some experimenting with your timing. Some people find a nice hot bath just before bed makes them drowsy and ready to drop into sleep. On the other hand, some people find that a hot bath is actually stimulating or that it makes them too uncomfortably warm when they slip into bed. If you find a just-before-bed bath makes it harder for you to fall asleep, consider taking the bath earlier, a couple of hours before bed. An earlier bath may enhance the gradual drop in body temperature that normally occurs at night and help trigger drowsiness.

4. MAKE YOUR BED A HAVEN

Most of us think of our bed as a place to sleep. But many people also use their bed for watching television, listening to the radio, talking on the telephone, eating, reading, or playing cards. If you really want to do all you can to sleep better, however, you shouldn't do any of these non-sleep activities in bed. When you do, the bed and bedroom can become associated with these activities rather than with sleep. Instead, you want to condition your mind and body to become drowsy and ready for sleep when you get into your bed, not ready and alert for a chat with a friend or a drama on TV. If you're one of those folks who sets the timer on the television or radio and drifts off listening to it, you might want to break yourself of the habit. You may not realize it, but you may be fighting off sleep just to hear the end of that monologue or the last bars of that favorite song. In addition, if you condition yourself to fall asleep only when you have that background noise, then if you wake up in the middle of the night, you may not be able to fall asleep without it. So you either struggle to fall back asleep without it or wake yourself up just to turn the device back on—neither of which is likely to improve your sleep overall.

5. STOP TRYING

While lying in bed, tossing and turning, you may become frustrated at your inability to slip into slumber. The more you try to will yourself into sleep, the more conscious you become of not being able to doze off.

But sleep is unlike most activities in life. While trying harder is often the surest path to success in business, sports, or other waking activities, it is the surest path to failure when you want to sleep. Sleep is most easily achieved in an atmosphere of total relaxation. Your mind should be empty of thought or turned to soothing and calming thoughts. Your body should be relaxed, your muscles free of tension. If you find you can't fall asleep, the best solution is to get out of bed. That's right. Contrary to popular belief, the solution is not to stay in bed. If this happens with any frequency, and you do stay in bed, you may begin to associate your room and bed with feeling frustrated, uncomfortable, and

unhappy. When you walk into your room, you'll immediately begin to worry about how long it will take to fall asleep.

Let your body associate any feelings of wakefulness with some other part of your home. Go to the kitchen for a drink of water. Go into another room and read, sew, or draw. Almost any activity will do as long as it's calming, relaxing, and doesn't require intense concentration. Gradually, you'll become tired and bored. Usually, within 15 to 20 minutes, your body will be ready for you to try to get to sleep again.

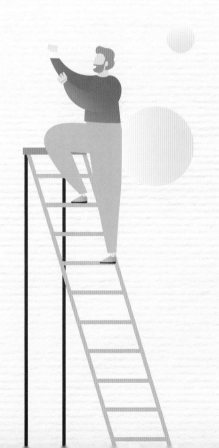

6. SNACK LIGHTLY BEFORE BED

If hunger pangs strike as you're preparing for bed, have a light snack. Research indicates that a light snack can help you sleep more soundly. The emphasis, of course, is on light. Bedtime is no time to stuff yourself. An overly full belly can be just as detrimental to sleep as an empty one would be.

Some researchers emphasize the importance of eating a nighttime snack that is high in carbohydrates, such as bread, potatoes, cereal, or juice. The carbohydrates, they contend, help usher tryptophan into the brain, where it is converted into serotonin. Some sleep scientists recommend eating foods that are rich in magnesium and/or calcium. These minerals have a calming effect on the nervous system, and even a slight deficiency of them, they say, can affect sleep. Dairy foods are good sources of calcium. Sources of magnesium include fruits such as apples, apricots, avocados, bananas, and peaches; nuts; and whole-grain breads and cereals. You might want to experiment with snacks from these various groups to see if they help you sleep.

7. ACTIVELY RELAX

An excellent way to quiet your body and mind before bedtime is to use one of the active relaxation techniques. These techniques help you to deliberately clear your mind of intrusive thoughts, wring the tension from your body, and put yourself into a peaceful state.

- Try progressive muscle relaxation (PMR). When you tense a muscle for a few seconds, it naturally wants to relax. That is how PMR works. You start at your toes and deliberately tense one muscle group at a time, progressively working your way up the body. To prepare, lie on your back on the floor or on a couch or recliner in a room other than your bedroom. Begin by scrunching your toes as hard as you can for ten seconds, while keeping the rest of your body relaxed. Then relax your toes, and tighten and release your calf muscles, again leaving your other muscles relaxed. Continue through the other muscle groups. Take your time at it; performing the muscle relaxation one time, from toes to head, should take at least 20 minutes. You should feel very relaxed when you finish. If you don't, repeat the entire cycle one more time.

- Try abdominal breathing. Rhythmic breathing is one of the best ways to help your body relax. There are many variations. This particular technique appears simple, but you'll need a little practice to do it properly. First, lie down on your back and begin to breathe normally. Now place your hand on your lower abdomen, just at your belt line, and slowly fill your lungs with air to the point that you can feel this portion of your abdomen rise. Take in as much air as you can and hold it for a couple of seconds. Then slowly release all the air in your lungs. Try to pay attention to nothing but the slow intake and release of air, the rhythmic rising and falling of your abdomen; don't rush. Repeat this eight to ten times.

◆ Try visualization. Imagine your favorite vacation spot. Maybe it's sitting on the sand with your bare feet being massaged by the ocean surf, or scuba diving off some coral reef. Alternately, think of an activity you find especially relaxing: drawing, cooking, hiking, walking your dog, even shopping. The idea behind visualization is to use your imagination to envision something that tells your mind to enjoy itself instead of being focused on some worry or concern.

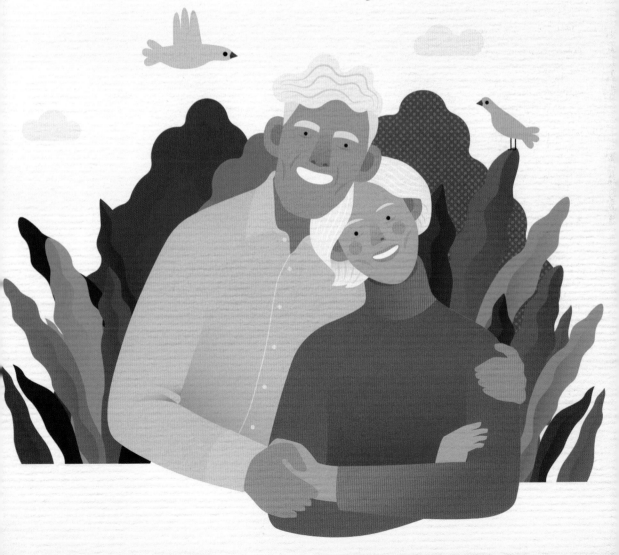

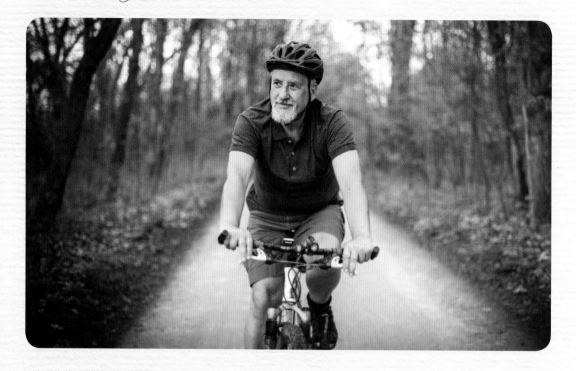

PROTECT YOUR HEAD FROM INJURY

Any discussion of the ways in which you can preserve youthful cognitive functioning as the years go by would not be complete without emphasizing the importance of shielding your brain from head injury and potentially toxic substances. Such assaults can cause lasting physical and cognitive damage.

If you want to make sure that your mind stays as sharp as possible for as long as possible, it's essential that you do all you can to avoid injury to your head. A growing body of research links head injury—especially the kind that causes traumatic brain injury (TBI)—to lasting and sometimes devastating problems with cognition, memory, and other brain functions. It is also linked to a higher risk of Alzheimer's disease and other forms of dementia. It makes sense to protect your head.

Awareness of the potential dangers of head injury has been growing in the United States. That increased attention is likely due at least in part to the expanding population of older Americans, who have an increased incidence of falls, as well as to the much-publicized struggles of several retired professional athletes who suffered traumatic brain injury from repeated head blows during their playing days.

Even a mild bump on the head can send the brain crashing into the bony cranium, disrupting normal brain function and causing TBI. TBI may be the result of direct physical damage to the brain as well as of a brief lack of oxygen flow to the brain cells, which prompts swelling inside the skull. Even what appears to be a very mild head injury can cause swirling movements throughout the brain, tearing nerve fibers and causing widespread blood vessel damage. Bleeding in the brain may cause even more damage. The temporal lobes of the brain appear to be especially sensitive to this kind of injury, so sensory and motor-control issues often accompany the cognitive, behavioral, and emotional problems that can result from TBI.

TBIs can range from mild to severe, depending on whether unconsciousness occurred and for how long; the severity of the symptoms caused by the TBI is also taken into account. A mild TBI, the kind that occurs most often, is commonly called a concussion and is not considered life-threatening. Loss of consciousness may not occur, but if it does, it lasts for no more than 30 minutes. Symptoms of a mild TBI can include confusion, dizziness, blurry vision, headache, ringing in the ears, nausea and vomiting, talking incoherently, changes in sleep or emotions, difficulty remembering new information, and an inability to remember what happened immediately before, during, and after the injury. Such symptoms may begin right after the injury or may only develop hours, days, or even weeks afterward, and they can last for months or even years.

A moderate TBI is one that causes loss of consciousness that lasts from 30 minutes to 24 hours, and a severe TBI causes unconsciousness lasting more than 24 hours. The symptoms of moderate and severe TBIs are similar to those of a mild one but their severity is increased. Both can be life-threatening. And both moderate and severe TBIs—as well as repeated blows to the head—can lead to a heightened chance of developing Alzheimer's disease and other types of dementia.

Among the top causes of TBIs are motor-vehicle accidents and falls. The best way to protect your head—and the rest of your body—from serious injury in a motor-vehicle crash is to wear your seat belt every time you are in a moving vehicle, no matter which seat you occupy or how short the trip.

Falls are the leading cause of TBIs, and they hit older individuals especially hard. More than 80 percent of TBIs in adults aged 65 and older are the result of falls. Falls also prompt the most hospitalizations for TBI in people 45 years of age and older. Aging can take a toll on eyesight, mobility, balance, and reaction time, increasing the risk of falls. To help keep you on your feet, try the following steps:

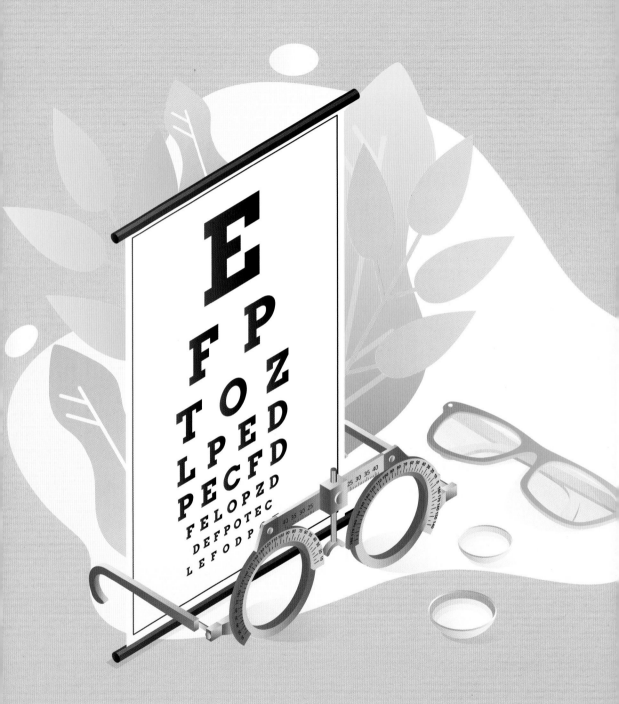

- Have your vision checked. If you're nearsighted, make sure your corrective lenses are up to date, and be sure to wear them. You have to be able to see obstacles in order to avoid them.

- Strengthen your legs with regular exercise. The leg muscles can grow weaker with age and leave you more vulnerable to falls.

- Avoid drinking alcohol. It affects balance, slows reflexes, and can leave you dizzy or sleepy.

- Review your medications with your doctor or pharmacist. Many over-the-counter and prescription medications can cause dizziness or light-headedness. Sleeping pills and heart and blood pressure drugs are among them. Taking multiple medications can aggravate the problem.

- Get rid of clutter in your home, especially on stairs, in hallways, and near doorways. It just creates obstacles for you to trip over.

- Wear well-fitting, low-heeled shoes with rubber soles both indoors and out. Stockings, socks, and slippers don't provide enough traction and can even make you more likely to slip. You might also want to skip open-backed shoes, which can slide off your feet as you're climbing stairs.

- Replace throw rugs that don't have skid-proof backs; if you can't, then make sure they are tacked down.

- Make sure every staircase has sturdy handrails and is well lit. Never try to go up or down stairs in the dark; even in the middle of the night, turn on the lights.

- Spread salt or even cat litter on icy walkways, stairs, porches, and driveways. And make sure these areas outside your home are well-lit at night; consider having motion-controlled fixtures installed.

- Make sure the rooms and hallways in your home are well-lit. Install more powerful bulbs or add lamps if necessary.

- Keep a flashlight next to your bed, and check it every so often to make sure it's in working order.

- Use nonstick mats in all tubs and showers, and install grab bars near the tub, shower, and toilet; consider getting a raised toilet seat.

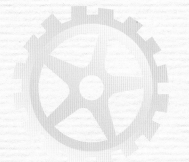

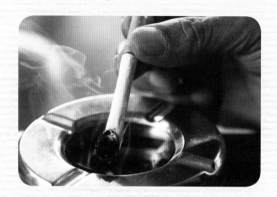

TOXINS

All your efforts to protect your brain from external blows will be for naught if you make lifestyle choices that assault your brain from within. And that's exactly what you're doing if you smoke cigarettes, abuse alcohol, or use illegal drugs. These toxins can stunt your brain's ability to withstand the passage of time.

If you're a smoker, puffing on that cigarette may make you feel reenergized—for a moment. But smoking can actually lower the amount of oxygen that reaches your brain, thereby affecting its functions, including memory and cognition. In fact, studies have found that smokers score lower on memory tests than do nonsmokers, and smokers who average more than a pack a day have an especially difficult time recalling names and faces. Some studies suggest that smoking can slow your recall ability about as much as having a couple of drinks. Smoking a pack a day exposes you to a variety of noxious substances, including 1,000 micrograms of toluene, which is highly toxic and can cause confusion and memory loss (as well as other damage). In other words, if you want to prevent premature brain (and body) aging, kick the habit. These days there are all sorts of products and programs that can help. Contact your doctor or local hospital to find out more.

Regularly having a few beers or glasses of wine (or a few of any alcoholic beverage) can begin to interfere with your brain function. Alcohol abuse destroys brain tissue and interferes with the process of absorbing information so that it never enters long-term memory. Indeed, short-term memory loss is often the first sign that alcohol-related neurological damage has occurred; it's also a hallmark of alcoholism. This type of memory loss means a person has difficulty remembering new information, so the learning process takes longer. Alcohol abuse also reduces higher-level thinking, or the ability to think in abstract terms, which is important for sound decision making, planning, and other abilities. If untreated, chronic alcohol abusers may even develop a form of dementia marked by disorientation, confused thinking, and severe amnesia. To put it plainly, excessive drinking actually changes the underlying brain chemistry that controls our abilities and skills. It can, and often does, threaten jobs and relationships. And it can certainly age your brain before its time. If you are struggling with alcohol, help is available. Contact your doctor or hospital for information about local programs and resources.

OUT OF IT

People who habitually drink too much may experience blackouts—periods of amnesia that occur when the amount of alcohol consumed prevents the formation of memories in the brain. Having a blackout is not the same as passing out. Indeed, they are not always marked by visibly altered states of consciousness. For example, a person may go out for drinks with friends and talk about work but then the very next morning not be able to recall that any such conversation even took place. How long blackouts last varies from person to person. But having them for any length of time is considered an early high-risk indicator of alcoholism.

RECREATIONAL DRUGS

When it comes to keeping your brain in tip-top shape no matter your age, there's no upside to dabbling in recreational drugs. The risk of lasting damage to your thinking and memory is simply too great. Marijuana, for example, can cause immediate as well as ongoing problems with short-term memory and attention. And both short-term and long-term use of opiates can negatively impact recall, reflexes, attention, concentration, hand-eye coordination, and executive functions. Recreational-drug use can even trigger symptoms that are similar to those of dementia.

PRESCRIPTION DRUG CAUTION

Some prescription medications can cause memory and cognitive problems. To avoid or minimize such effects:

- Show your doctor a list of everything you take, including prescription and over-the-counter medications, vitamins and minerals, supplements, and herbs.

- Fill all of your prescriptions at the same drugstore, so that the pharmacist can spot potential drug interactions, including those that can cause memory or cognitive problems.

- Never combine medications (even over-the-counter ones) with alcohol.

- Take your medicines exactly as prescribed. Never double a dose without your doctor's or pharmacist's approval, even if you missed the previous dose.

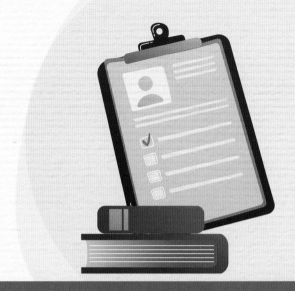

HONING YOUR MEMORY

Have you ever walked out of a mall and completely forgotten where you parked your car? If it happened to you when you were 20 years old, you probably didn't think anything of it. Once you're in your fifties and sixties, however, you may begin to wonder if such memory gaps are simply due to aging—or something worse.

But no matter your age, occasionally forgetting where you parked your car or where you left personal items is often completely normal. It's known as "everyday forgetting," and it's so common because it involves things we do every day and usually don't spend much time paying attention to. And that lack of attention is the very reason these instances of everyday forgetting occur.

Of course, as you get older, you're more likely to think—and worry—about memory problems. And the more you worry about them, the more likely you are to notice each and every slip. Odds are you forgot quite a few things when you were in your teens and twenties, but you never paid much attention to those lapses, and you certainly didn't worry about them. The fact is, the more you expect to have memory problems, the more you'll notice them.

The best way to stop this vicious circle is to focus on remembering instead of forgetting. Rather than expending mental energy fretting about every little memory slip, you need to pay more attention to the act of remembering. Once you begin to do this, you'll be amazed at how much better your memory will be.

REMEMBER HOW MEMORY WORKS

Your baby's first cry . . . the taste of your grandmother's molasses cookies . . . the scent of an ocean breeze. These are memories that make up the ongoing experience of your life. They're what make you feel comfortable with familiar people and surroundings, tie your past with your present, and provide a framework for the future. In a profound way, it is our collective set of memories—our "memory" as a whole—that makes us who we are.

Most people talk about memory as if it were a thing they have, like bad eyes or a good head of hair. But your memory doesn't exist in the way a part of your body exists—it's not a "thing" you can touch. It's a concept that refers to the process of remembering. In the past, many experts were fond of describing memory as a sort of tiny filing cabinet full of individual memory folders in which information is stored away. Others likened memory to a neural supercomputer wedged under the human scalp. But today, experts believe that memory is far more complex and elusive than that—and that it is located not in one particular place in the brain but is instead a brain-wide process.

Do you remember what you had for breakfast this morning? If the image of a big plate of fried eggs and bacon popped into your mind,

you didn't dredge it up from some out-of-the-way neural alleyway. Instead, that memory was the result of an incredibly complex constructive power—one that each of us possesses—that reassembled disparate memory impressions from a web-like pattern of cells scattered throughout the brain. Your "memory" is really made up of a group of systems that each plays a different role in creating, storing, and recalling your memories. When the brain processes information normally, all of these different systems work together perfectly to provide cohesive thought.

What seems to be a single memory is actually a complex construction. If you think of an object—say, a pen—your brain retrieves the object's name, its shape, its function, perhaps even the sound when it scratches across the page. Each part of the memory of what a "pen" is comes from a different region of the brain. The entire image of "pen" is actively reconstructed by the brain from many different areas. Neurologists are only beginning to understand how the parts are reassembled into a coherent whole.

If you're riding a bike, the memory of how to operate the bike comes from one set of brain cells; the memory of how to get from here to the end of the block comes from another; the memory of biking safety rules from another; and that nervous feeling you get when a car veers dangerously close, from still another. Yet you're never aware that these are separate mental experiences nor that they're coming from all different parts of your brain, because they all work together so well. In fact, experts tell us there is no firm distinction between how you remember and how you think.

This doesn't mean that scientists have figured out exactly how the system works. They still don't fully understand exactly how you remember or what occurs during recall. The search for how the brain organizes memories and where those memories are acquired and stored has been a never-ending quest among brain researchers for decades. Still, there is enough information to make some educated guesses. The process of memory begins with encoding, then proceeds to storage, and eventually moves to retrieval.

ENCODING

Encoding is the first step in creating a memory. It's a biological phenomenon, rooted in the senses, that begins with perception. Consider, for example, the memory of the first person you ever fell in love with. When you met that person, your visual system likely registered physical features, such as the color of their eyes and hair. Your auditory system may have picked up the sound of their laugh. You probably noticed the scent of their perfume or cologne. You may even have felt the touch of their hand. Each of these separate sensations traveled to the part of your brain called the hippocampus, which integrated these perceptions as they were occurring into

one single experience—your experience of that specific person. Experts believe that the hippocampus, along with the frontal cortex, is responsible for analyzing these various sensory inputs and deciding if they're worth remembering. If they are, they may become part of your long-term memory. As indicated earlier, these various bits of information are then stored in different parts of the brain. How these bits and pieces are later identified and retrieved to form a cohesive memory, however, is not yet known.

Although a memory begins with perception, it is encoded and stored by nerve cells using the language of electricity and chemicals. The connections between nerve cells in the brain aren't set in concrete—they change all the time. Brain cells work together in a network, organizing themselves into groups that specialize in different kinds of information processing. As one brain cell sends signals to another, the synapse between the two gets stronger. The more signals sent between them, the stronger the connection grows. Thus, with each new experience, your brain slightly rewires its physical structure. In fact, how you use your brain helps determine how your brain is organized. It is this plasticity that can help your brain rewire itself if it is ever damaged.

As you learn and experience the world and changes occur at the synapses and dendrites, more connections in your brain are created. The brain organizes and reorganizes itself in response to your experiences, forming memories triggered by the effects of outside input prompted by experience, education, or training.

These changes are reinforced with use, so that as you learn and practice new information, intricate circuits of knowledge and memory are built in the brain. If you play a piece of music over and over, for example, the repeated firing of certain cells in a certain order in your brain makes it easier to repeat this firing later on. The result: You get better at playing the music. You can play it faster, with fewer mistakes. Practice it long enough and you will play it perfectly. Yet if you stop practicing for several weeks and then try to play the piece, you may notice that the result is no longer perfect. Your brain has already begun to forget what you once knew so well.

To properly encode a memory, you must first be paying attention. Since you cannot pay attention to everything all the time, most of what you encounter every day is simply filtered out, and only a few stimuli pass into your conscious awareness. If you remembered every single thing that you noticed, your memory would be full before you even left the house in the morning. What scientists aren't sure about is whether stimuli are screened out during the sensory input stage or only after the brain processes its significance. What we do know is that how you pay attention to information may be the most important factor in how much of it you actually remember.

EASIER ENCODING

If you want to remember a word, thinking about how it sounds or its meaning will help. Likewise, if you use visual imagery to help memorize something —such as meeting a person named Mr. Bell and thinking of a bell when you shake hands—you're more likely to remember it. Some experts believe that using imagery helps you remember because it provides a second kind of memory encoding, and two codes are better than one.

MEMORY STORAGE

Once a memory is created, it must be stored (no matter how briefly). Many experts think there are three ways we store memories: first in the sensory stage; then in short-term memory; and ultimately, for some memories, in long-term memory. Because there is no need for us to maintain everything in our brain, the different stages of human memory function as a sort of filter that helps to protect us from the flood of information that we're confronted with on a daily basis.

The creation of a memory begins with its perception: The registration of information during perception occurs in the brief sensory stage that usually lasts only a fraction of a second. It's your sensory memory that allows a perception such as a visual pattern, a sound, or a touch to linger for a brief moment after the stimulation is over.

After that first flicker, the sensation is stored in short-term memory. Short-term memory has a fairly limited capacity; it can hold about seven items for no more than 20 or 30 seconds at a time. You may be able to increase this capacity somewhat by using various memory strategies. For example, a ten-digit number such as 8005840392 may be too much for your short-term memory to hold. But divided into chunks, as in a telephone number, 800-584-0392 may actually stay in your short-term memory long enough for you to dial the telephone. Likewise, by repeating the number to yourself, you can keep resetting the short-term memory clock.

Important information is gradually transferred from short-term memory into long-term memory. The more that you repeat or use the information, the more likely it is to eventually end up in long-term memory, or be "retained." (That's why studying helps people to perform better on tests.) Unlike sensory and short-term memory, which are limited and decay rapidly, long-term memory can store unlimited amounts of information indefinitely.

People tend to more easily store material on subjects they already know, since the information has more meaning to them and can be mentally connected to related

information that is already stored in their long-term memory. That's why someone who has an average memory may be able to remember a greater depth of information about one particular subject. Most people think of long-term memory when they think of "memory" itself—but most experts believe information must first pass through sensory and short-term memory before it can be stored as a long-term memory.

TYPES OF REMEMBERING

Psychologists have identified four types of remembering.

RECALL: This is what you most often think of as "remembering"—the active, unaided remembering of something from the past.

RECOLLECTION: This is the reconstruction of events or facts on the basis of partial cues, which serve as reminders.

RECOGNITION: This is the ability to correctly identify previously encountered stimuli—such as when you see your old teacher's face across the room and recognize who she is.

RELEARNING: This type of remembering is a testament to the power of the memory itself; material that's familiar to you is often easier to learn a second time.

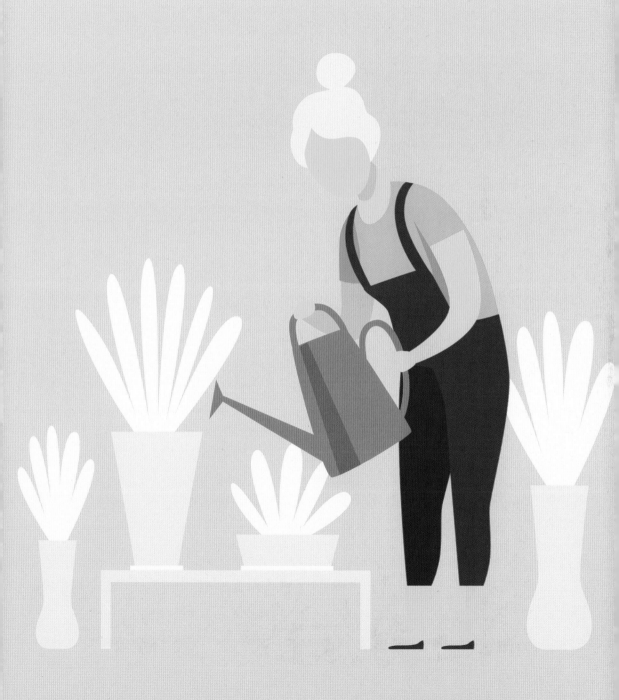

MEMORY RETRIEVAL

When you want to remember something, you retrieve the information on an unconscious level, bringing it into your conscious mind at will. While most people think they have either a "bad" or a "good" memory, in fact, most people are fairly good at remembering some types of things and not so good at remembering others. If you do have trouble remembering something—assuming you don't have a physical disease—it's usually not the fault of your entire memory system but an inefficient component of one part of your memory system.

Let's look at how you remember where you put your eyeglasses. When you go to bed at night, you must register where you place your eyeglasses: You must pay attention while you set them on your bedside table. You must be aware of where you are putting them, or you won't be able to remember their location the following morning. Next, this information is retained, ready to be retrieved at a later time. If the system is working properly, when you wake up in the morning you will remember exactly where you left your eyeglasses.

If you've forgotten where they are, you may not have registered clearly where you put them. Or you may not have retained what you registered. Or you may not be able to retrieve the memory accurately. Therefore, if you want to stop forgetting where you left your eyeglasses, you will have to work on making sure that all three stages of the remembering process are working properly.

If you've forgotten something, it may be because you didn't encode it very effectively, because you were distracted while encoding should have taken place, or because you're having trouble retrieving it. If you've "forgotten" where you put your eyeglasses, you may not have really forgotten at all—instead, the location may never have gotten into your memory in the first place.

Distractions that occur while you're trying to remember something can really get in the way of encoding memories. If you're trying to read a business report in the middle of a busy airport, you may think you're remembering what you read, but you may not have effectively saved it in your memory.

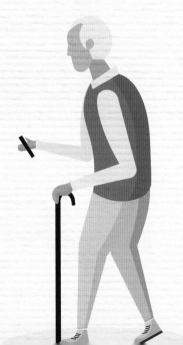

Finally, you may forget because you're simply having trouble retrieving the memory. If you've ever tried to remember something one time and couldn't, but then later you remember that same item, it could be that there was a mismatch between retrieval cues and the encoding of the information you were searching for.

You'll be better able to remember something if you use a "retrieval cue" that occurred when you first formed a memory. If you memorized a poem outdoors when birds were singing, then playing birdsong might help you recall the poem. This is why vivid memories will recur strongly when you experience a sensation that accompanied the original event. It's why, for example, the sound of a car backfiring may trigger an unpleasant memory of a battlefield experience for someone who was previously in a war zone.

AGE GAP

Research suggests that older people have some trouble with all three stages of memory, but they have special problems with registering and retrieving information.

SIGNS OF SOMETHING MORE

The following are common warning signs that memory problems may be more than everyday forgetfulness and therefore should warrant a medical evaluation:

- Memory problems that affect job performance or interfere with everyday functioning

- Difficulties with language, such as frequently forgetting simple words or substituting inappropriate words

- Disorientation in familiar locales or in familiar situations

- Confusion about time of day, month, season, or decade

- Decreased or unusually poor judgment

- Memory problems accompanied by other symptoms such as extreme fatigue, loss of interest in activities that are typically enjoyed, rapid or unusual changes in mood, agitation, listlessness, problems with balance or coordination, headaches, vision problems, numbness, shortness of breath, or chest pain.

It's important to keep in mind that there are a variety of factors that can cause memory problems, such as stress, vitamin deficiencies, and circulatory problems; not all memory problems signify the onset of Alzheimer's disease. That's why a thorough medical evaluation is needed when memory problems are out of the ordinary or prompt concern. Once the underlying cause is determined, it can often be treated, and the memory problems remedied as a result.

PAY ATTENTION!

Everyday forgetting is linked to the fact that when you've done something so many times in the past, it can be hard to remember if on this particular day you've turned off the stove. Indeed, some people go through entire routines of "checking" in the morning because they know they have problems remembering if they've actually turned off appliances and closed windows before leaving for the day.

If you really want to cure such everyday absentmindedness, you need to become acutely aware of what you're doing. When you don't pay attention, you're not likely to register information in the first place. The likely result: forgetting. Paying attention takes effort. There may be times when your attention strays—think of the times you've rushed out the door because you were running behind schedule, only to discover later that you left behind something important. Instead, you need to slow down and focus on one thing at a time.

It is important to concentrate on what you are doing, especially when it comes to things you're not usually good at remembering. For example, have you ever been driving to work and tried to remember whether or not you unplugged the iron? To improve your ability to remember such everyday occurrences, you need to pause and pay attention as you turn off or unplug an appliance so that it will register in your memory. This helps to turn an automatic act into a conscious one.

HERE ARE THE STEPS:

1. Before going out the door, stop and take the time to think. If you're locking your back door, think about what you're doing.

2. Focus your concentration. Speak out loud to force yourself to pay attention. If you often forget to turn off the stove, go into the kitchen and force yourself to slowly survey the appliances. As you look at each one, say "The oven is turned off. The toaster is unplugged." When you're driving down the road and you ask yourself if the oven is off, you'll know that it is.

3. Go over everything. If you tend to leave important things behind, create a list of them, and line them all up before you leave. Go through each item, saying it out loud. Check your calendar to assure yourself that everything you need is lined up and ready.

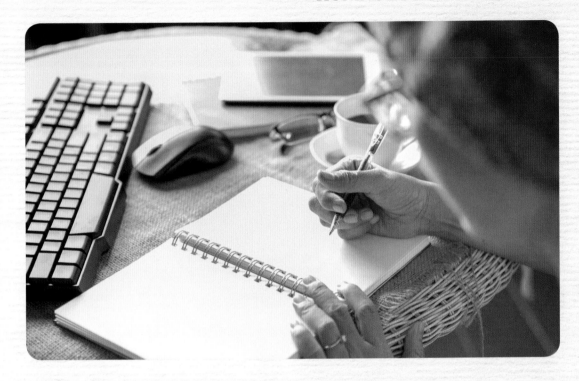

4. Take immediate action. Do you need to take back that library book? Do it now, while you're thinking about it. At least put the book by the front door; lean it right up against the door if you have to.

If you're plagued by a bit of general absentmindedness, it could mean that your life is simply a bit out of control. You're most likely to be absentminded when you're preoccupied. Those who are easily distracted or who tend to be daydreamers are particularly vulnerable to interference.

Here's a quick list of ways to regain some control over your daily life and your memory:

1. Get organized. Develop a routine and stick to it. If you're organized, you can often make up for not remembering certain things by keeping information and various possessions in easily accessible places.

2. Make lists. Keep a daily to-do list, and cross off items once they've been done. Always keep the list in the same place, and organize the list into categories. Make your list easy to find: Put it on a large, colored sheet of paper.

3. Keep a calendar handy to keep track of important dates. Check the calendar at the same time every day so it becomes a habit. When you buy a new calendar at the beginning of the year, transfer all important dates from the old calendar.

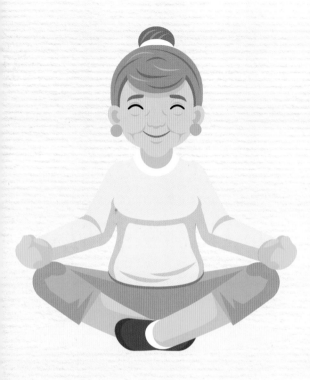

7. Make visual cues: Place a colored sticky note on your steering wheel, protruding up from your briefcase or purse, or on your bathroom mirror, your shoes, or your wallet. Don't assume you'll remember; leave reminders.

8. Keep important numbers in one place, so you can locate them even if you're under a lot of stress. Be sure to keep critical numbers (phone numbers, medical insurance, etc.) in your wallet.

9. Write things down as they occur—use lists, schedules, and so on. If you use a smart phone or tablet, type them into the device.

10. Return items that you frequently use to the same spot each time, and rely on placement to trigger your memory (for example, leave an umbrella on the doorknob).

4. Have a place for everything, and put everything in its place. If you have a key rack right inside your door, you'll be more likely to hang your keys there and remember where they are.

5. If you need to remember to take certain things to work or school, keep a tote bag or backpack right by the front door. Keep all papers and items that need to go with you in that bag or backpack.

6. Concentrate on one thing at a time, and try to pay active attention each time you put something down.

11. Repeat yourself. If someone tells you information that you need to remember, repeat it over and over again to yourself.

12. Keep a positive attitude about memory lapses as you get older. Remember, memory decline is not inevitable. Be sensitive to the many things that can make you prone to forget. You can take action to overcome or mitigate most of them. Even when memory lapses cause you some aggravation, try not to dwell on them. If you constantly tell yourself that you have a bad memory, it may become a self-fulfilling prophecy.

WORK ON WEAK SPOTS

Not all aspects of memory slow down as we age. And whether young or old, some people are simply better at remembering certain things, like names, while other folks are good at recalling dates or directions. It is unrealistic to expect to remember everything. But you can get better at remembering those things that you aren't—and perhaps have never been—good at remembering. The following are strategies that you can employ to get better at remembering specific types of information.

REMEMBERING HABITUAL TASKS

If you have trouble remembering habitual tasks such as turning off the coffee pot each morning or feeding the cat, the key to solving this problem is to relate the activity to something that you don't generally forget to do every day. For example, if you often forget to take your medication in the morning, tell yourself each day that you won't eat your breakfast until you have taken your pill. Make swallowing that pill a prerequisite to taking your first bite of food. By incorporating a task into an outline of things that you don't forget to do, you will be less likely to forget that task. You can even make the connection a physical one, say by storing your bottle of medication right in front of your cereal box in the cabinet.

RECALLING WHERE YOU PUT THINGS

There is hope for those who can't remember where they left their car keys or their purse. The main reason you forget where you put these items is because you weren't paying attention when you put them down. Because you weren't paying attention in the first place, when it comes time to retrieve the memory of where you left the object, you can't. It was never properly absorbed into your short-term memory in the first place.

The solution is really quite simple: Pay attention. And if you can't pay attention, be consistent. Make a concerted effort to pay attention to where you are placing the keys. Stop yourself in the middle of dropping them on the desk and take a deep breath. Stare at the desk and say out loud, "I am putting my keys on the desk."

If you force yourself to pay attention, you're less likely to forget when it comes time to retrieve that particular memory. The other sure-fire way to remember particular items is to put them back in exactly the same place, every single time. Find specific places to keep all the items that are often misplaced:

- Glasses
- Keys
- Medications
- Coupons
- TV remote
- Cell phone

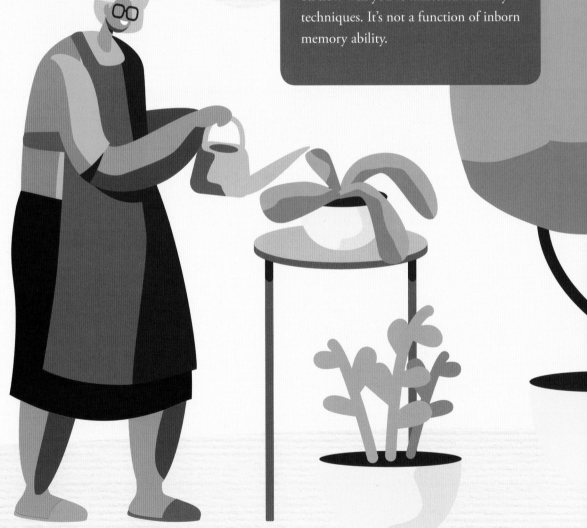

MEMORY MYTH

MYTH: I just have a bad memory and there's nothing I can do about it.

FACT: Remembering is a learned skill. It can be developed just like any other skill. In the absence of disease, the strength of your memory depends on how well you've mastered memory techniques. It's not a function of inborn memory ability.

REMEMBERING YOUR SCHEDULE

It won't matter much if you can remember to do something in the future if you don't remember to do it at the right time. For example, you may remember that you need to mail in your IRS payment a week before the deadline, but if you forget all about the task on the day you intended to do it and the deadline subsequently passes, you haven't solved your problem. In fact, a problem with remembering dates is one of the most common memory failures. A combination of mental strategies and mechanical reminders should help get this problem under control.

One way to solve the problem of forgetting dates is to cue your attention. For example, you could take your IRS payment and tape it to the front door, or tape a dollar bill to the front door to remind yourself. Here are some tried-and-true cues:

- Attach a safety pin to your sleeve.

- Put a rubber band around your wrist.

- Move your watch to the opposite arm.

- Leave a note to yourself (a brightly colored sticky note is ideal) in a prominent place.

- Set a reminder on your cell phone, tablet, or computer—but only if you use it every day.

Using a calendar is an excellent mechanical method of remembering dates. The key is not to use two calendars—one at home and one at work. Get one calendar that's convenient to carry with you. Or, if you use a smart phone or can access your computer both at home and at work, try using the device's calendar program to keep track of appointments and important dates electronically. Whatever calendar you ultimately choose, all important days should be marked down. Every morning, consult the calendar and cross off items as they occur. On the first day of the new year, get out a new calendar and transfer all of the important dates from the old calendar so you don't forget anything.

REMEMBERING WHAT YOU'RE DOING

We've all gone into a room and totally forgotten what we're doing there. If you've done this, you're not alone; experts suggest that more than half of all Americans experience this problem. It's not incipient dementia; it's just a lack of attention.

Each time you have a thought about going into a room to get something, stop for a moment and tell yourself out loud what you are going to get. If you're already in the other room and can't remember what you're doing there, try retracing your steps to where you were standing when you had the thought to leave the room. This form of association will often help jog the memory of your errand.

REMEMBERING PLACES

It's not unusual to forget where you've parked the car. Here's how to remember where you parked it: After you park your car in a big parking lot, don't just get out of the car and head straight for your destination. Stop. Look around and make a mental note of where you are. Find something that will help you remember: Did you park next to a tall lamp post? Is there a parking number or letter posted to help you find your way? Check to see if there's a sign on the store or in the store window that aligns with the row you parked in, and repeat what the sign says to yourself as you enter the store. Better yet, write a description of the location on the parking garage ticket or other paper and put it with your keys. Don't rely on a description of the cars parked around you; they could very well be gone when you come back for your car.

If you tend to lose your way as you walk, ride your bike, or travel in a car, you need to better register the way as you go:

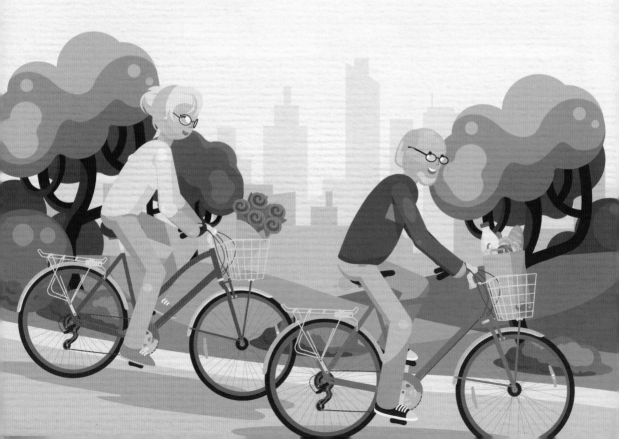

- As you travel, try to take mental snapshots along the route. Flash back to them in your mind once in a while.

- Record visual "cues" from both directions if you can (things might look different from the opposite direction). Look for that big red barn, the funny sign, the crooked tree.

- Use all your senses. Pay attention to unusual smells or noises; the more senses you involve, the stronger the memory trace will be.

- Use GPS or maps. If your phone or car does not have GPS and you're not good at reading maps, write down directions, study them thoroughly before you leave, and bring them with you.

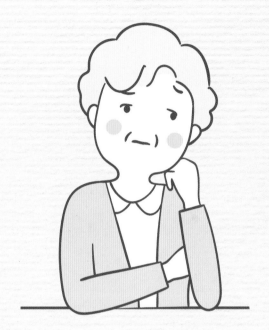

If all else fails and you have a really hard time finding your car, try making it stand out: Attach a brightly patterned flag, a lightweight rubber toy (like a squeaky toy), or a neon table tennis ball to the tip of your car's antenna. This way, you'll have a better shot at spotting your vehicle from a distance. You might also consider parking further out in the lot, where there tend to be fewer vehicles parked to begin with, so it's easier to pick out your car from a distance.

REMEMBERING QUANTITIES

If you've ever been in the midst of baking brownies and suddenly realized you have no idea how much flour you've dumped in the bowl, you need help in paying attention to amounts. Try visualizing the amount of flour in the measure. Pour it in while saying out loud the amount you're using, "One cup, two cups . . . " You'll find that when you comment out loud on how many cups you've put in, you're less likely to forget or get sidetracked.

You may want to resort to a backup strategy. For every cup of flour you pour, set aside an object to represent that cup: a coffee bean, a raisin, a spoon. Each time you add another cup of flour, set aside another bean or raisin. This way you can visually check exactly how much you've added, even if you're continually interrupted.

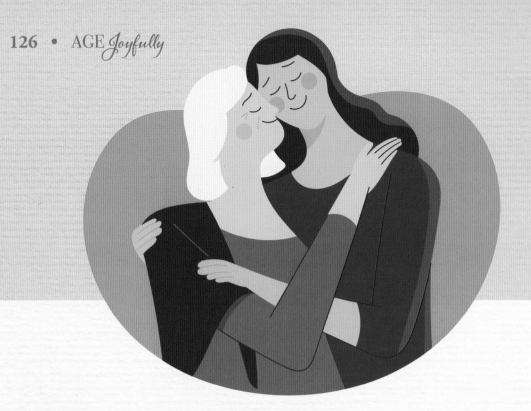

REMEMBERING NAMES

There you are at a business party, chatting with someone whose name you've forgotten. A third person comes up and you're expected to make an introduction, but you can't remember the name.

This is certainly not unusual. Most of us can remember faces quite easily, even if we've only seen them once or twice. But when it comes to attaching a name to that face, that's another matter entirely. We tend to remember faces more readily because it involves the process of recognition, whereas attaching a name to the face requires a process called recall. What's the distinction? Recognition is much easier for the brain to accomplish, because recognition simply requires you to choose among a limited number of alternatives that are present in front of your eyes—sort of like a multiple-choice question. But to recall a name, the brain has to go digging for it, which is a much more complex process. Recall, then, is more like a fill-in-the-blank question.

The process of recall is generally easier if we have some retrieval cues that give the brain some direction. One way to do this is to associate an individual's name with another piece of information that you already know. For example, when you first meet a person and hear their name, you might tell yourself that this person has the same name as your mother-in-law or the same name as your favorite baseball player.

You can also use the verbal technique to help implant a person's name in your memory when you first meet them. **To do this, simply:**

1. Register the person's name: Pay attention to it as it is said!

2. Repeat the person's name to yourself.

3. Comment on the name.

4. Use the person's name out loud as soon as possible.

Another strategy for remembering names is to use the visual technique. **There are three simple steps to get the name right every time using this technique:**

1. Associate the name with something meaningful. That's easy with a name like "Bales" (picture two bales of hay). If it's something more difficult, like Sokoloff, think of "Soak it all off" and picture a giant sponge sopping up spilled milk.

2. Note distinctive features of the person's face.

3. Form a visual association between the face and the name. If you've just met Jill Brown, and she has very dark eyes, picture those brown eyes as you say the name to yourself.

After you've done all you can to remember the name, you need to rehearse the name if you're going to remember it. Repeat the name to yourself again in about 15 seconds. If you've met several people, repeat the names to yourself while picturing the faces before the end of the event. The more often you can repeat the names early on, the more likely they will stick in your head. Remembering names can be an important social skill; we all like to think that other people remember us. The ability to remember names of even slight acquaintances is highly regarded.

RECALL VS. RECOGNITION

Trying to answer the following questions can help you understand the difference between recognition and recall.

RECALL
Who was the president of the United States during the Civil War?

RECOGNITION
Who was president of the United States during the Civil War?

A) Benjamin Franklin

B) Abraham Lincoln

C) John Quincy Adams

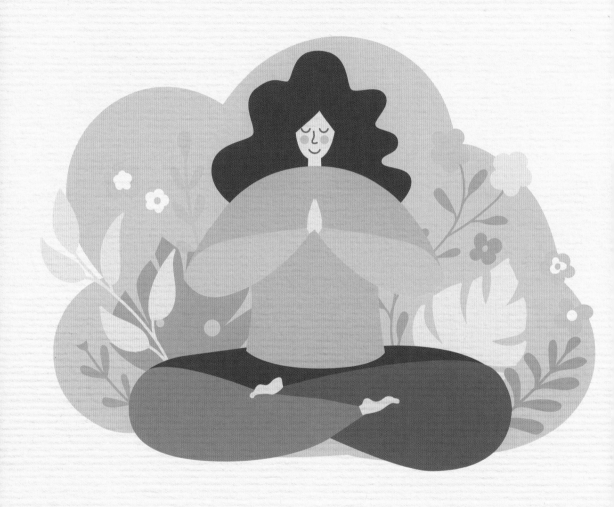

THE NAME GAME

Here's one way to practice remembering names. Cut out ten magazine photos, each showing a person's face. Enlist a partner, give that person five of the photos, and keep the remaining five photos for yourself. Write a name on each of your five photos (pick five random names—preferably not the names of your children or your five best friends), and ask your partner to do the same with their five photos. Now exchange photos, and practice trying to associate the name with something distinctive about the person's face. Wait about 15 minutes, then quiz each other on the names.

EXERCISE YOUR MIND

You can improve your mind at any age. And many experts agree that one of the best ways to keep your mind sharp—or improve it if it's starting to show some signs of age—is to exercise it throughout your life.

We've all heard that getting regular physical activity can keep your heart muscle strong and flexible. And we explored how physically moving your body's muscles can help protect your brain. Well, even though your mind is not a muscle, it, too, needs regular mental exercise to perform the way it should year after year. One great way to exercise your mind and keep it nimble is to continually stimulate it with new and interesting experiences and opportunities to learn. Another is to challenge it with a wide range of puzzles, riddles, games, and activities that allow it to stretch its proverbial legs and run. These forms of mental calisthenics will prompt the creation and activation of more connections between nerve cells as well as the birth of new nerve cells in cognitively important areas of the brain. The more numerous and active your brain-cell connections and the faster they become at sending signals back and forth, the better your mind will work.

STIMULATING A BETTER BRAIN

Modern neuroscience has established that our brain is a far more elastic organ than was previously thought. In the past it was believed that an adult brain could only lose nerve cells (neurons) and couldn't acquire new ones. Today we know that new neurons—and new connections between neurons—continue to develop throughout life, even well into advanced age. Thanks to recent scientific discoveries, we also know that we can harness the powers of plasticity to protect and even enhance our minds at every stage of life—including our advanced years. Recent scientific research demonstrates that the brain responds to mental stimulation much like muscles respond to physical exercise. In other words, you have to give your brain a workout. The more vigorous and diverse your mental life the more you will stimulate the growth of new neurons and new connections between neurons. Furthermore, the nature of your mental activities influences where in the brain this growth takes place. The brain is a very complex organ with different parts in charge of different mental functions. Thus, different cognitive challenges exercise different components of the brain.

Thanks to MRI and other sophisticated imaging technologies, we know that certain parts of the brain grow in size in people who use these parts of the brain more than most people do. For example, in one study, researchers found that the hippocampus, a major player in spatial memory, was larger than usual in London cab drivers who were required to remember and navigate complex routes in the huge city. Other studies have revealed that Heschl's gyrus, a part of the brain's temporal lobe that is involved in processing music, is larger in professional musicians than in musically untrained individuals. And the angular gyrus, the part of the brain involved in language, proved to be larger in bilingual people than in those who speak only one language.

What is particularly important about these findings is that the size of the effect—the extent to which the part of the brain was enlarged—was directly related to the amount of time each person spent in the activities that rely on the part of the brain in question. For instance, the hippocampal size was directly related to the number of years the cab driver spent on the job, and the size of Heschl's gyrus was associated with the amount of time a musician devoted to practicing a musical instrument. Enlargement of a brain region indicates a greater than usual number of neurons and synapses. What these research findings show, therefore, is that our behavior directly influences and changes the structure of the brain. The impact of cognitive activity on the brain can actually be great enough to result in an actual increase in its size!

It is also true that any more or less complex cognitive function—be it memory, attention, perception, decision making, or problem solving—relies on a whole network of brain regions rather than on a single region. Therefore, any relatively complex mental challenge will engage more than one part of the brain, yet no single mental activity will engage the whole brain.

For this reason, it is important to have a rich, challenging, and diverse mental life. The more vigorous and varied your cognitive activities, the more efficiently and effectively they'll protect your mind from decline. To return to the workout analogy: Imagine a physical gym. No single exercise machine will make you physically fit. Instead, you need a balanced and diverse workout regimen. The same is true for your brain.

EXPAND YOUR MIND'S HORIZONS

As long as you stay active, interested in life, and engaged in the world around you, your memory and other cognitive abilities don't have to deteriorate as you grow older. Research shows that enriching your surroundings, your daily experiences, and your life as a whole can pay off in a sharper, more resilient mind.

For example, animal studies have found that rats living in cages with plenty of exciting toys and lots of stimulation have larger, healthier brain cells and a larger outer brain layer. Deprived rats living in barren cages, on the other hand, have smaller brains.

Research in humans strongly indicates that stimulating the brain in a variety of ways throughout life can help to protect cognitive function. It also appears to provide a kind of mental reserve that helps delay signs of normal brain aging as well as loss of cognitive function related to Alzheimer's disease and other types of dementia.

What can you do to enrich your brain's environment? Get out and see new places, meet new people, and experience new things. **For example:**

- Take up a new hobby or sport.

- Visit museums, art galleries, or historical sites in your area that you've never previously taken time to explore.

- Take a class at a community college, or go back to school and get the degree you've always wanted.

- Check out listings for free lectures or seminars at your local library, civic center, or senior center, and attend those that pique your interest.

- Join a volunteer organization or a book club.

- Investigate your ancestors and plot out your family tree.

- Track down old friends and find out what's been happening in their lives since you last communicated.

- Make sure you have music playing for at least a little while every day; while any music is good, research has found that classical music is especially stimulating to the intellect.

- Keep lots of books on hand, and make time to read them. If you can't block out specific reading times, keep a paperback in your purse or briefcase or download a book to your tablet or e-reader so you can squeeze in some reading while you're riding a train or bus or waiting for an appointment.

- Add a fish tank to your home or office with lots of colorful fish and interesting tank toys.

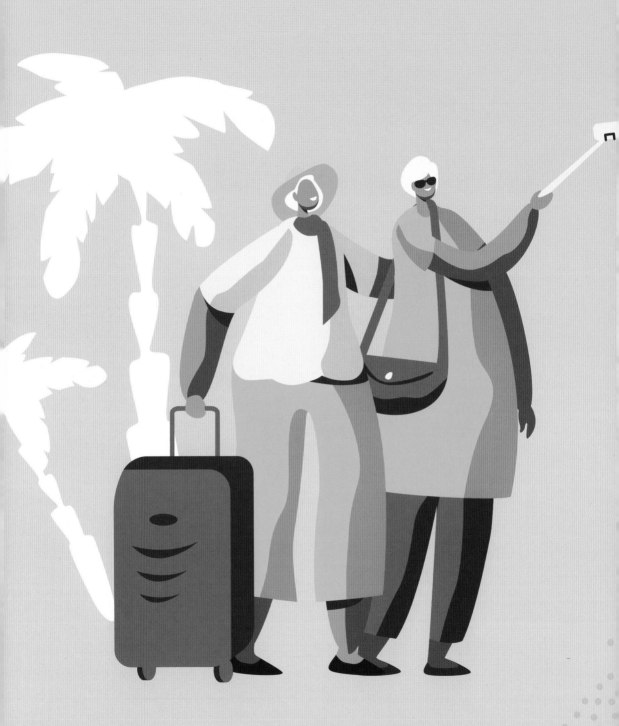

◆ Paint the walls of your home interesting, unusual colors. Select interesting art, knickknacks, rugs, and curtains. Try to include a variety of textures with things like pillows, blankets, and furniture fabrics.

◆ If you have the space, put a birdhouse and a bird feeder or birdbath outside your window, and keep a pair of binoculars handy. Add some brightly colored flowers to your yard or place planters or window boxes outside your windows.

◆ Don't forget the flowers indoors, too; the colors and smells will be an added sensory boost.

◆ Set out a jigsaw puzzle or chessboard and regularly engage visitors in a game.

◆ Plug in a computer and use it to surf the Internet or play a challenging game; computer games can improve memory in such fun ways you'll hardly notice the effort.

◆ Try cooking food from a different culture, or visit restaurants with cuisines that are not usually on your menu.

◆ Include others in your life. Some research indicates that strong social connections can help stave off depression and Alzheimer's disease and keep you alert and interested in life. Make an effort to spend time with other people, especially if you do not have relatives or close friends nearby. Get to know your neighbors by inviting them over for a cup of coffee or glass of lemonade. Attend some of the various get-togethers held at your house of worship so you can meet other congregants. Keep an eye out for interesting social activities and gatherings or volunteer opportunities in your area and use them as ways to meet potential new friends. We'll talk more about this in the next chapter.

Remember, anything that engages the senses will help to stimulate your mind and strengthen your memory. So touch, feel, smell, and experience new things as often as you can.

PICTURE THIS!

Visualization is another good exercise for your brain. Try to visualize something from your childhood: your bedroom in the house where you grew up, your first-grade classroom, the inside of your parents' car when you were a teenager. Visualization helps stimulate the mind and exercise the brain cells. If you picture a happy or comforting place from your past, visualization can also serve as a relaxation tool by giving you a pleasant mental detour away from worries.

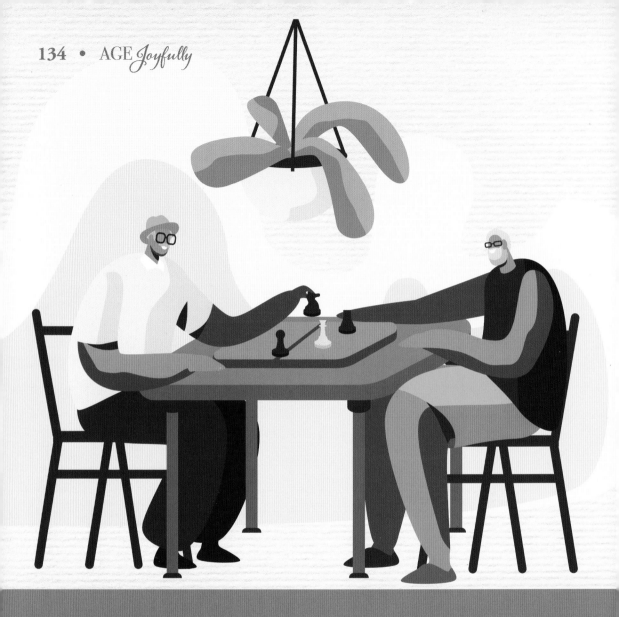

STAYING CONNECTED

What does playing bingo have to do with staying healthy? It's not the temporary increase in heart rate when you jump up to shout "bingo!" And it's not the money you may take home after an evening of card games, either. It's the social aspect of game playing that is good for you. Staying socially connected and engaged turns out to be an elixir of life.

WITH A LITTLE HELP FROM FRIENDS

Being active and involved feels good, but it's more than a mood booster—not that there's anything wrong with that! Getting out there and doing things actually helps protect you from the kind of physical problems that can decrease your independence. Recent research shows that seniors who ate at restaurants occasionally, traveled (day trips or longer), participated in community groups, went to sports events or religious services, and visited friends were the least likely to be disabled later in life.

In fact, socially active people were twice as likely as those who are not very active to be disability-free as they aged. They were better at taking care of themselves and were more physically mobile.

Whether you see yourself as an outgoing person or are more the quiet type, your connections with family and friends are precious—and not just because they make you happier and more contented. Your social connections help keep you mentally sharp and physically healthy.

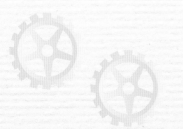

CONNECTING VIA THE WORLD WIDE WEB

Are you wired? That's the term used to describe people who take advantage of the Internet.

The computer and other new technology keep you connected with family, friends, and community resources in very important ways:

E-mail lets you write to and receive messages from those near and dear to you quickly—and even in real time if you use an instant-messaging feature.

E-mail also lets you receive and send photographs. There's no waiting for the kids to get photos printed and mailed—which could be never! Is your granddaughter pregnant? You can follow the expansion of her belly with the frequent photographs she e-mails to you.

Free computer-to-computer long-distance phone services like Skype not only let you talk to people via the Internet, they let you see those people too! If, like increasing numbers of grandparents, you live some distance from your grandchildren, you can visit with them every day if you want via Skype. Even if the children and grandchildren lived closer, you might not see them in person as often as you are able to visit with them virtually.

Some of the latest cell phones have video-chatting and video-conferencing capabilities. That means you can be in touch with friends and family wherever they (or you) roam.

Facebook lets you keep up to date with family members unobtrusively—and there's an immediacy to it that is hard to duplicate. It turns out to be an especially valuable way to connect with and even become close with the grandkids. If they accept you as a friend on Facebook—which many will do even if they don't "friend" their own parents—you can follow their daily (sometimes hourly!) postings and status updates, see their most recent photographs, and get a sense of their lives and what's on their minds.

GETTING TECHNICAL

If you haven't already joined the Internet generation or your skills aren't up to snuff, there are lots of places to get help learning the ropes. Here are some to get you started:

- Ask a friend or relative (especially grandchildren—it's another opportunity for bonding!) who is computer savvy to teach you.

- Take a free or low-cost computer class locally. Libraries, community colleges, park districts, community centers, senior centers, and local government offices (such as cities or suburbs, townships, and counties) often offer beginning computer classes for older adults. Check them all out to find the least expensive, most convenient classes.

- If you don't own a computer, you will find free computers to use at libraries and at senior or community centers.

- Contact your local Area Agency on Aging. You can call the Eldercare Locator at **800–677–1116** or visit **www.eldercare.gov.**

E-MAIL ETIQUETTE AND PROTECTION

Where's Amy Vanderbilt when you need her? New rules of etiquette have developed for writing and sending e-mail messages, and there are also some important safety rules. These are some basics so you don't inadvertently send the wrong message or leave yourself vulnerable to cyber attacks.

- Do not write in all capital letters. This is considered akin to shouting or yelling at the recipient. (DO NOT USE ALL CAPS—see, doesn't that feel like the letters are screaming at you?).

- Log out of your e-mail account when you are not using it. This is especially important if you are using a public computer, such as those at a library, community center, or even a store. Your e-mail is protected by a password, but if you don't sign out, anyone who uses the computer next could access your e-mail—putting you at risk for identity theft and all kinds of mischief using your personal information.

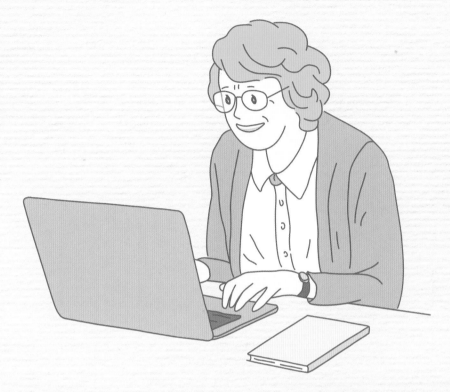

• If you're sending an e-mail to many people, not just to a small circle of friends or relatives who know each other, list all the e-mail addresses in the BCC (Blind Carbon Copy) field instead of in the To or CC field. That way you are not sharing everyone's e-mail addresses with strangers.

• Do not accept your computer's invitation, via a pop-up message, to "remember your password." You may be prompted frequently to do that, but although it may seem convenient, it is actually quite dangerous. If the computer remembers your password for you, then anyone who opens it has access to your e-mail—and through it to other personal information.

FRIENDS INDEED

Want to predict how you'll feel after you retire? Count the number of friends you have, not how much money you squirreled away or how healthy you are.

That's right: The most powerful predictor of post-retirement happiness is the size of your social network, said a University of Michigan study. The researchers could even give the happiness factor a number: 16. Study participants who said they were "most satisfied" with life had an average of 16 people in their social networks. Those who were least satisfied had networks of fewer than 10 people.

The results stand to reason, since retirement can shrink the amount of daily interaction you have with people and leave you feeling isolated. Having a solid group of good friends will provide the emotional support you need to negotiate the life changes that come with retirement. Even if you're ecstatic about retirement, it is still a significant life event—and positive changes cause stress, too, as you adjust to the new normal.

FRIENDSHIP
SILVER AND GOLD

Friends understand your life in a way that family does not. And they can be a buffer when family troubles create tough times. Most of all, friends are fun.

What to do if you come up several friends short of the magic number in your social network?

1. Be a good friend—to those you already have and to acquaintances you may not have put yourself out for before. Strengthen all the relationships you have.

2. Be on the lookout. Join clubs and organizations or participate in activities and events in which you are interested. Keep your eyes open for someone interesting to talk with who shares your passions.

3. Reconnect with old friends. Everyone loses touch with old friends over the years while working and raising families, so don't let embarrassment get in your way. This is the perfect time to get reacquainted—and to reminisce. Even if a significant number of years have passed, old friends will feel comfortable immediately.

4. Start using social networking tools like Facebook and Twitter. These will take you in directions that you may not be able to imagine. From finding former schoolmates to meeting people with similar health issues, social networking sites have the capacity to expand your universe exponentially.

5. Make friends with people who are younger than you are. Younger friends can bring energy to your life and fill in the holes left by friends who are absent due to moves, illness, or even death.

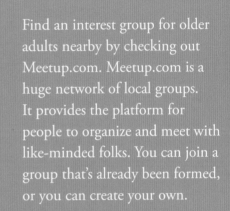

Find an interest group for older adults nearby by checking out Meetup.com. Meetup.com is a huge network of local groups. It provides the platform for people to organize and meet with like-minded folks. You can join a group that's already been formed, or you can create your own.

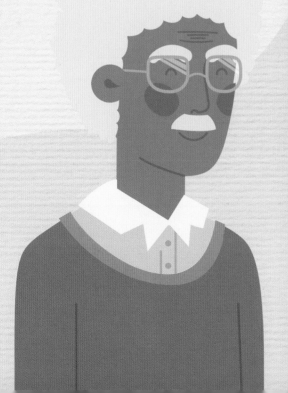

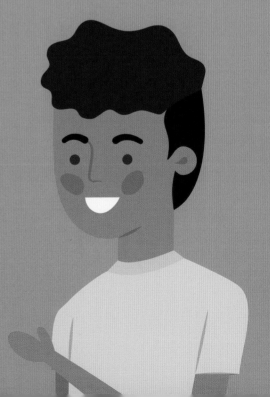

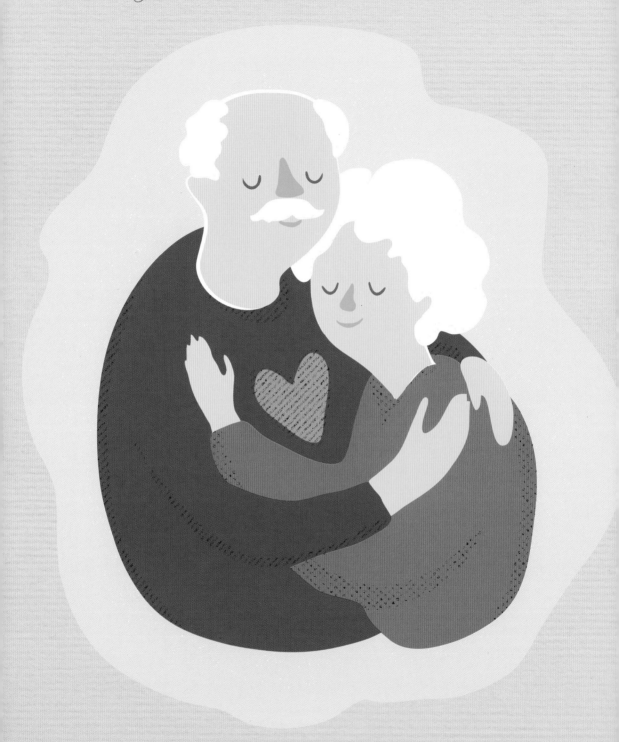

DATING AND ROMANCE

If you're a single senior, you've got plenty of company. According to the U.S. Census Bureau, about 46 percent of Americans older than age 65 do not have a partner. Millions of older Americans are widowed, divorced or separated, or were never married.

Some seniors are quite happy to be on their own, but many are looking for someone with whom to share and enjoy life. Companionship is a priority. Love and romance would be great, of course, though not all seniors are necessarily interested in marriage. Whatever your desires and dreams, it takes some effort to seek and find a person you can care about and who cares for you.

Before you put a toe in the dating waters, though, be sure you're ready. If you have lost a partner through death or divorce, ask yourself a few questions before jumping into the dating game:

- Are you past the emotions of the previous relationship?

- Do you feel you have to tell your life story on the first date?

- Are you ready to listen to the other person?

- Are you ready to have fun?

One dating expert suggests that you make a short list of what you are looking for in a partner. There is a good chance you're looking for different traits than you wanted when you were dating in your teens and twenties.

ONLINE DATING

It's not easy for seniors to meet someone to date or to find a potential new partner. That's why many are taking their cues from younger singles and trying their luck on the Internet. Some of the popular sites are www.match.com and www.eharmony.com. There is even a dating site just for people over 50 called OurTime.com.

When you go online, you might be able to browse the prospects a bit without signing up, but at some point early on, you will be asked to fill out a personal profile before you will be allowed access to more. And sooner or later you'll need to pay a fee, as these sites all charge for continued access and usage. If you do sign up, you'll want to include a picture, so start looking for one that puts your best face forward. Or ask a friend to take a new photo of you to post. One expert suggests taking a picture of yourself doing something you enjoy.

Once you find someone who looks interesting, get acquainted first by e-mail and then by phone. When you're ready to meet in person, choose a public place, such as a coffee shop or restaurant.

Remember, there are charmers out there who are looking to rip you off. Until you know your new love really, really well, be cautious.

- Make the first dates in the daytime and for short amounts of time—just for coffee, for example.

- Don't give out your home phone number or your home address. This allows you to guard your personal information until you get to know the person well.

- When you're going to meet someone, always let friends or family know where you are going and when.

- Watch out for anyone who might want to borrow money or get information about your bank account.

- Do not leave your purse or wallet open or unattended.

- Keep your drink, no matter what kind it is, near you, and don't leave it unguarded to avoid tampering.

- Don't drink alcohol. It may relax you, but it will also cloud your judgment and relax your inhibitions. You want to be clear-headed and in control on the first several dates at least.

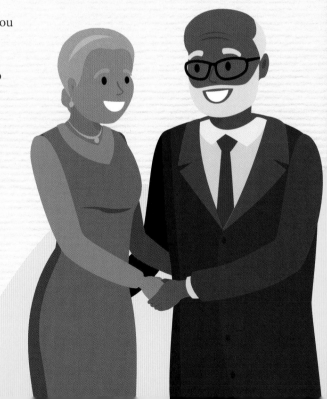

If you are thinking of getting a pet, make sure it fits your lifestyle. This is not the time to take on a big, strong, demanding animal. Instead consider adopting a mature cat or dog who is past the rambunctious stage and won't take over your home.

If you can't adopt a pet, you can get your strokes in and reap the health benefits by volunteering at a local animal shelter. Grooming, petting, and playing with furry friends are therapeutic activities, even if the pets aren't yours.

PET POWER

Do you share your home with a special animal? If a pet is part of your life, then you are taking care of more than a Fido or Fluffy. You are taking care of yourself!

Research shows that pets help people live longer and better lives. Pet owners get over illnesses more quickly and have lower blood pressure and cholesterol levels than non-owners, and they need to visit the doctor less frequently.

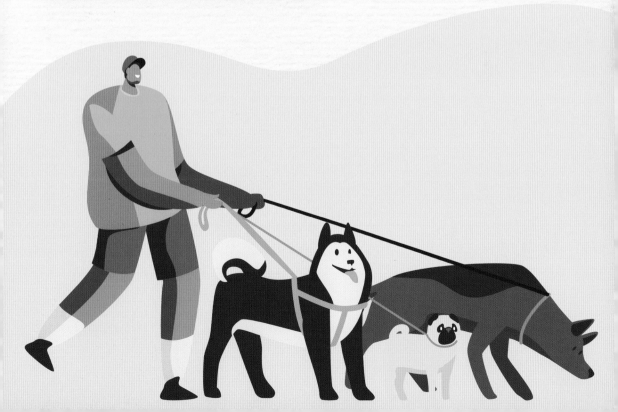

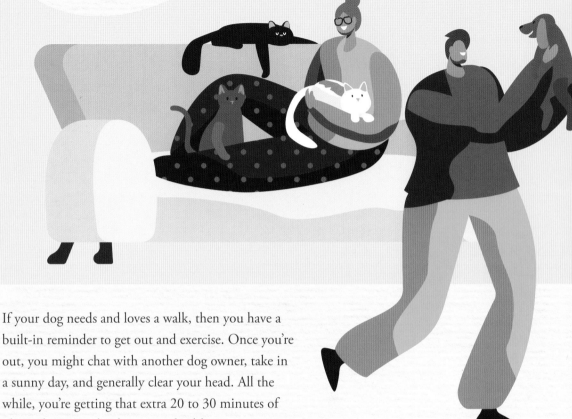

If your dog needs and loves a walk, then you have a built-in reminder to get out and exercise. Once you're out, you might chat with another dog owner, take in a sunny day, and generally clear your head. All the while, you're getting that extra 20 to 30 minutes of physical activity that keeps you healthy.

Your dog or cat loves you for yourself, not because you're wearing the latest fashion. A pet's unconditional love is a powerful antidepressant. If petting your dog or cat makes you feel good, it's not an accident. It's scientific. Cuddling with your four-legged pal releases endorphins, hormones that help you relax.

So who cares if there's a little pet hair sticking to your nice black slacks?

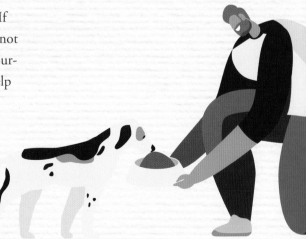

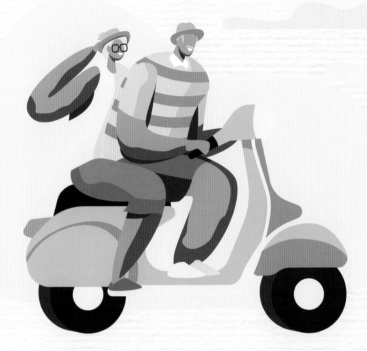

BUILDING COMMUNITY

We are part of many different kinds of communities during our lives, but where we live is the most obvious and has the most impact. As we get older our communities change, and so do our needs and desires. We leave some communities, such as our workplace, and need to build connections to new ones. People who feel connected are happier and healthier.

It used to be that senior citizens only had a few options when it came to housing: living independently in a home or apartment, or moving to an assisted living or nursing home situation that felt more like a human warehouse than a home or community.

Today, there are many more possibilities. A whole spectrum of housing options have been developed—and more continue to be developed—so that you truly can pick a living arrangement that fits your personality, your budget, and your needs and also fosters the connections that are so critical to your long-term health and satisfaction.

Here are some newer living options to consider that you may not know about:

In **cohousing communities**, residents may have the best of both worlds: independence and strong community life. Residents live independently, usually in a single-family detached home, a townhome, or a condo apartment, but share common spaces that encourage social contact. There is a common house that functions as a social center and includes a dining room and kitchen for optional group meals several times a week, recreational spaces, and other amenities. Decisions about allocation of dues are made together as a community, and residents meet regularly to socialize, to solve problems, and to develop community policies. Cohousing communities are sometimes designed with input from future residents, and the homes are clustered to promote contact with neighbors and for proximity to the common house.

For more information about cohousing, visit the Cohousing Association online at www. cohousing.org.

One new type of community, **Village to Village,** helps older people with the low-cost support they need to stay in their own homes. It's an "aging in place" model, which many seniors prefer. The first village started in Boston in 2001, and now there are at least 56 villages in the United States—with more than 120 in the works.

Here's how it works: Members pay a reasonable yearly fee, which entitles them to services that run the gamut from home repairs to transportation to health and wellness programs to social and educational activities. Villages are run by volunteers and paid staff.

For more information, visit **www.vtvnetwork.org.**

The standard **continuing care retirement community (CCRC)** offers different levels of health care on one campus, so you can obtain increasing amounts of assistance as you need it without having to move to a new community or residence. Generally there is a one-time entrance fee and then monthly premiums for a wide range of other services, such as nursing care, housekeeping, meals, and social programming.

A newer version of a CCRC is the Continuing Care at Home (CCAH) program, which is a more affordable alternative that allows you to remain in your own home while receiving services such as care coordination and routine home maintenance, in-home caregivers, transportation, meals, and wellness programs. With a CCAH, you can develop your own personalized care plan. CCAH programs are sometimes operated by nonprofit organizations. To find information about CCAHs in your area, contact your local or state's department of aging.

Homesharing is another creative way to remain in your home, lower your costs, and have a source of companionship. You share your home with an unrelated person who needs a place to live. There are many match-up programs across the country; some only function as referral services while others offer matching services and follow-up throughout the homesharing relationship.

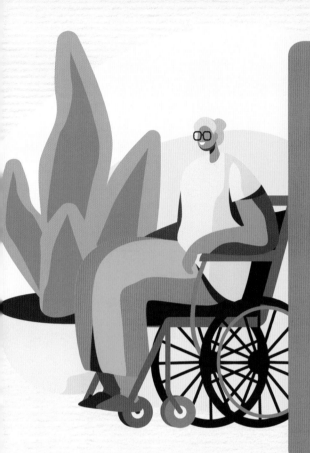

SCAM ALERT!

What will the scammers think of next? Con artists are now calling seniors claiming to be a grandchild in need. They say they're traveling and need $500 sent by way of Western Union right away. If this happens to you, do these things before you panic and send cash:

- Check with the parents, even if the "grandkid" said to keep it a secret.

- Ask personal questions that only the real grandchild would know how to answer.

- Call the police.

ADAPTING YOUR HOME

Aging in place is a great idea, but what if your current residence isn't so user-friendly as you get older? An industry has sprung up with specialists trained to help people age 50 and older alter their homes to meet their changing needs.

The Certified Aging in Place Specialist is a designation developed by the National Association of Home Builders Remodelers Council, in collaboration with AARP, the NAHB Research Center, and the NAHB Seniors Housing Council, to give professionals the skills they need to serve the older adult population. Certified aging-in-place specialists (CAPS) are trained to modify homes and provide solutions to common problems that seniors confront in their daily lives. These changes can be as simple as adding grab bars to the shower or tub area and lever door handles in place of knobs to make them easier to open. Other common remodeling improvements are widening doorways to accommodate a wheelchair and installing elevated sinks and dishwashers to reduce bending and back strain.

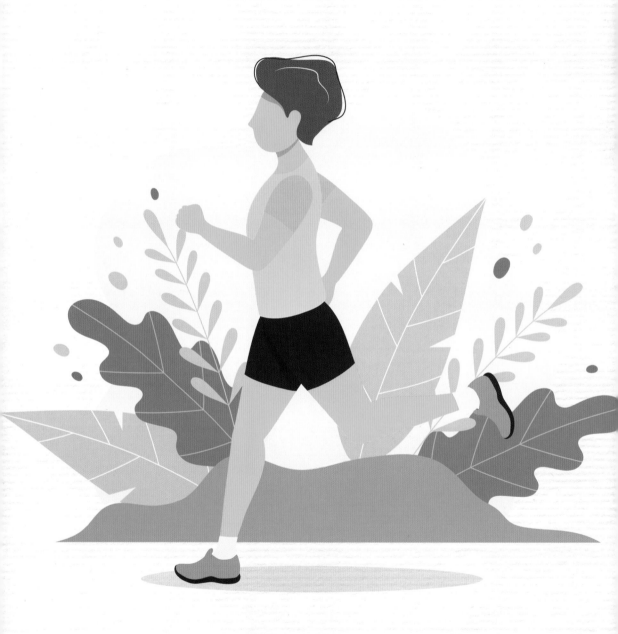

FIT AND FLEXIBLE

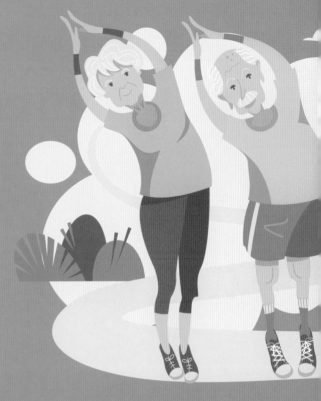

We've talked about the importance of exercise and movement in this book, and for good reason. Exercise combats a variety of health conditions: heart disease, high blood pressure, elevated blood sugar, diabetes, elevated cholesterol, depression, and increased stress. It protects your brain against Alzheimer's. It burns extra calories, an important added benefit for those who need to lose weight. Physical activity also produces chemical messengers called endorphins that help relieve anxiety and pain.

Being physically active every day is as much a state of mind as it is a state of being. It means taking every opportunity to move more. The simple act of walking more may be enough to start setting things right. A wearable fitness tracker can work wonders. When you incorporate exercise into your daily routine, the activity or activities that you choose should also be something that you enjoy, that you have easy access to, and that is safe and reasonable for you to perform given your current health, abilities, and schedule. Your selection also needs a thumbs-up from your doctor, especially if

you haven't been active lately. Most people who have had a relatively sedentary lifestyle find that low-impact activities such as walking and swimming are perfect. In this chapter, you'll find step-by-step instructions and accompanying photographs for:

- Cardiovascular exercises to keep your heart and lungs healthy

- Strength-training exercises to challenge your muscles

- Yoga exercises for flexibility and balance

CARDIO EXERCISES

MARCH IN PLACE

Marching in place is a low-intensity, moderate-impact exercise. Like other cardio activities, it increases the heart rate to strengthen the heart and lungs while also increasing circulation throughout the body. If neuropathy of the feet is present, do seated.

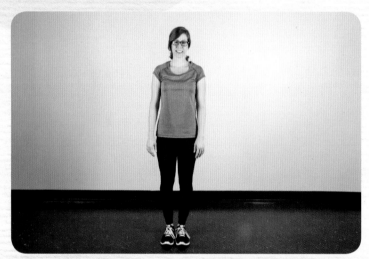

STEP 1

Stand (or sit) tall with abdominals pulled in.

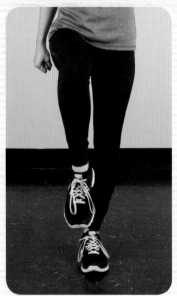
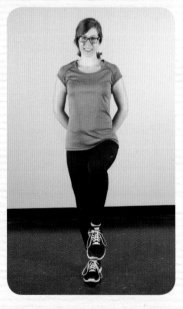

STEP 2

March in place for 1–2 minutes.

STEP 3

For added intensity,
swing arms.

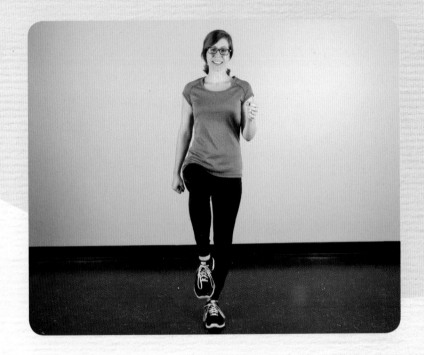

RUN IN PLACE

Running in place is a moderate-intensity, moderate-impact exercise. Avoid this exercise if neuropathy of the feet is present.

STEP 1

Stand tall with
abdominals pulled in.

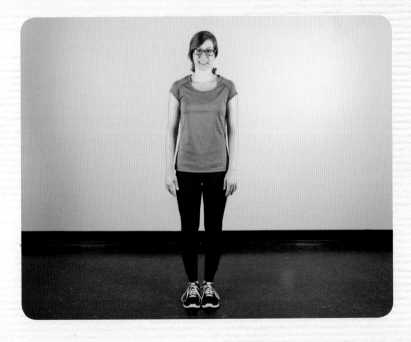

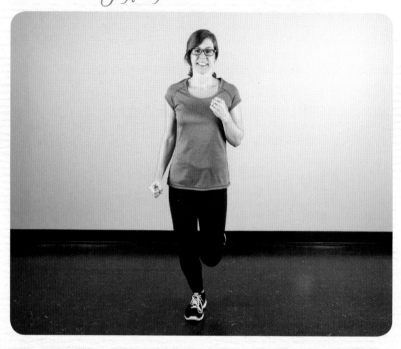

STEP 2

Run in place for
1–2 minutes.

STEP 3

For added intensity,
swing arms.

HEEL TAPS

Heel taps are a low-intensity, low-impact exercise. Along with providing cardiovascular benefits, heel taps also aid in stretching the back of legs and ankles.

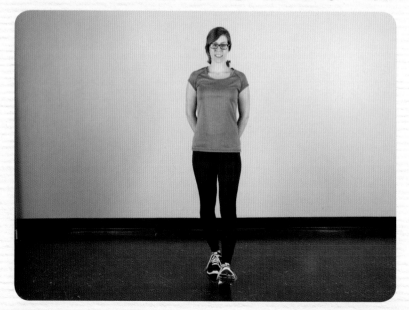

STEP 1

Stand (or sit) tall with
abdominals pulled in.

Using a quick pace,
alternating legs,
tap heels on floor
for 1–2 minutes.

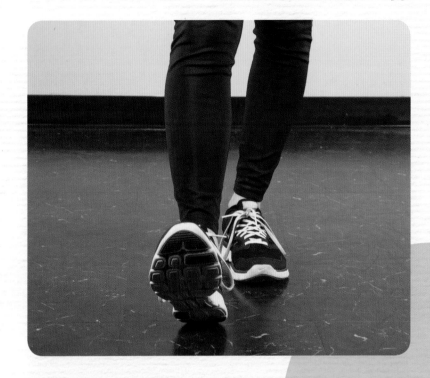

STEP 2

As you do this exercise, keep toe pointed to ceiling.

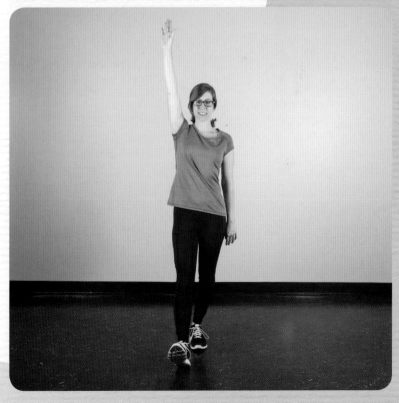

STEP 3

For added intensity, add an arm reach to ceiling.

TOE TAPS

Toe taps are a low-intensity, low-impact exercise. Along with providing cardiovascular benefits, toe taps also aid in stretching the front of legs and ankles.

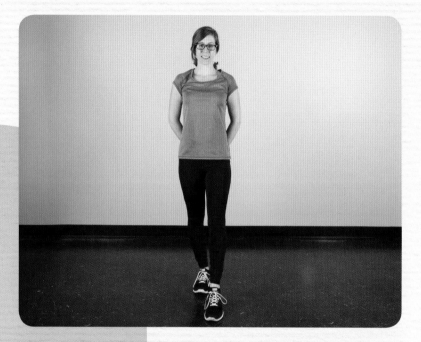

STEP 1

Stand (or sit) tall with abdominals pulled in.

Using a quick pace and alternating legs, tap toes on floor for 1–2 minutes.

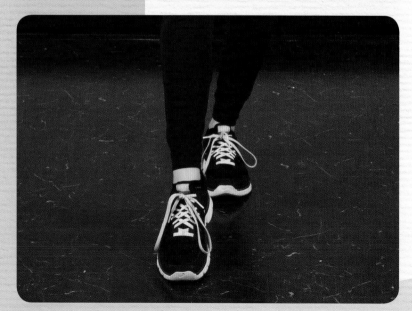

STEP 2

As you do this exercise, keep toe pointed to floor.

STEP 3

For added intensity, add an arm reach to ceiling.

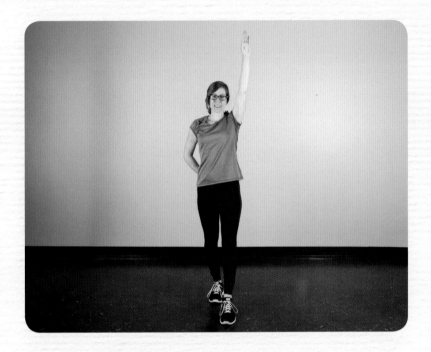

JUMP ROPE

Jumping rope is a moderate-intensity, high-impact exercise. This can be done with a rope or by twirling the arms without a rope. If neuropathy of the feet is present, do this exercise in a chair, omitting the rope.

STEP 1

Stand (or sit) tall with abdominals pulled in.

Begin to hop in place, twirling arms forward or using a jump rope. Hop for 1–2 minutes.

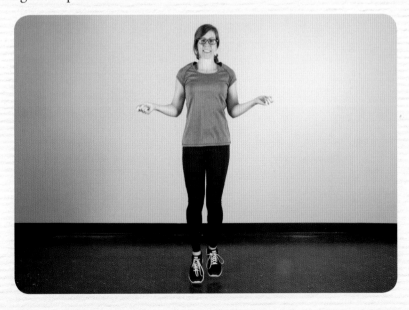

HIGH KNEES

High knees are a moderate-intensity, moderate-impact exercise. Along with providing cardiovascular benefits, high knees also aids in strengthening the hip and core muscles. If neuropathy of the feet is present, do seated.

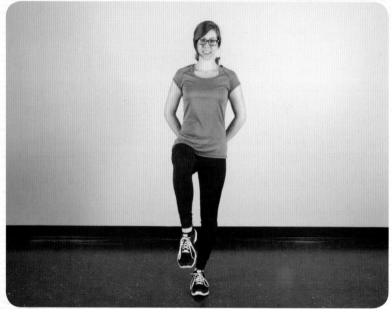

STEP 1

Stand (or sit) tall with abdominals pulled in.

Alternating legs, pull knees to hip level.

STEP 2

As you do this exercise, keep spine straight. Lift knees for 1–2 minutes.

STEP 3

For added intensity, add a forward press with arms.

SIDE STEPS

Side steps are a low-intensity, moderate-impact exercise. Along with providing cardiovascular benefits, side steps strengthen the outer and inner thighs. If neuropathy of the feet is present, do seated.

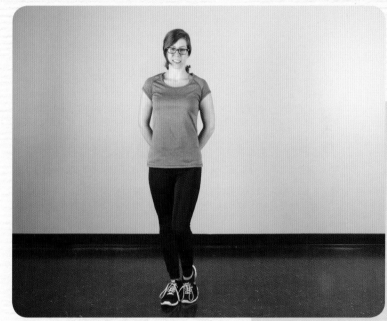

STEP 1

Stand (or sit) tall with abdominals pulled in.

Step both feet to the left and then step both feet to the right.

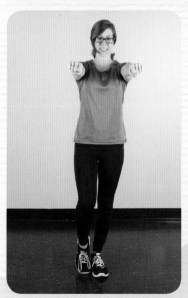
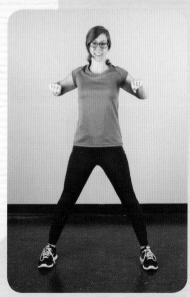

STEP 2

Step side to side for 1–2 minutes.

For added intensity, add a pulling movement with arms.

FORWARD AND BACK STEP

Stepping forward and back is a low-intensity, moderate-impact exercise. Along with providing cardiovascular benefits, stepping forward and back aids in training the walking and balance muscles of the upper leg. If neuropathy of the feet is present, do seated.

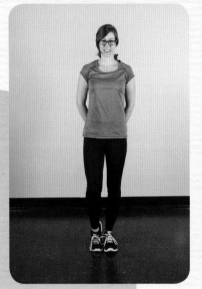
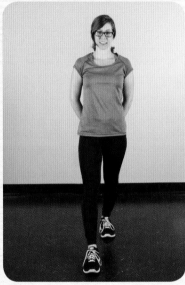

STEP 1

Stand (or sit) tall with abdominals pulled in.

Step both feet forward.

STEP 2

Step both feet back. Step forward and back for 1–2 minutes.

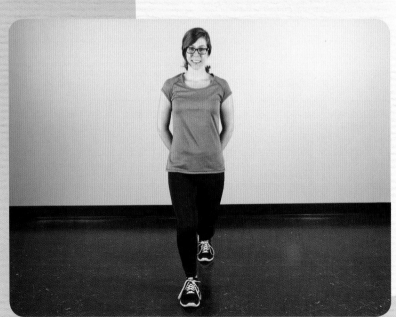

STEP 3

For added intensity, add a knee bend with the forward step.

JUMPING JACKS

Jumping jacks are a high-intensity, high-impact exercise. If neuropathy of the feet is present, modify exercise or do seated.

STEP 1

Stand (or sit) tall, abdominals pulled in.

Jump feet out to either side while bringing arms up overhead. Then return to start. Jump for 1–2 minutes.

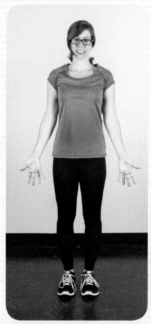
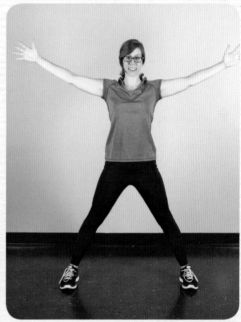

STEP 2

To modify, alternate side taps with feet while bringing arms up over head.

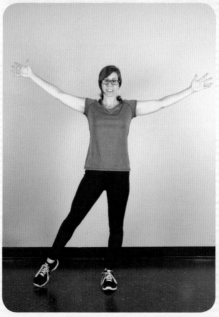
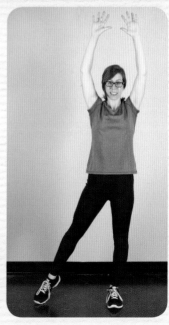

STRENGTH EXERCISES

BICEP CURLS

Bicep curls are a low-intensity, no-impact exercise. This exercise strengthens the front of the arm, the muscle used for lifting and rotating the arm outward.

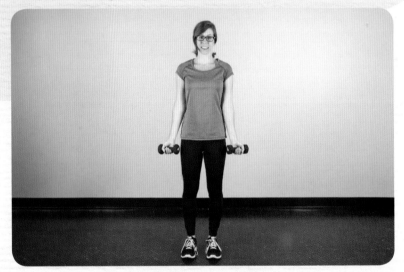

STEP 1

Stand (or sit) tall, feet at hip distance.

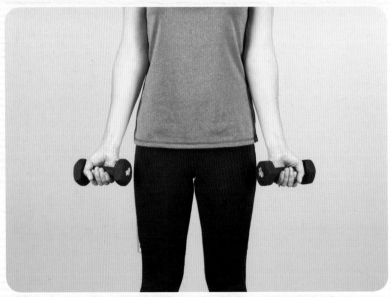

STEP 2

Put arms straight down by sides, palms facing up.

STEP 3

Keeping the elbows close to ribs, curl hands up towards shoulder.

STEP 4

The exercise can be done with one or both arms. Do 10–15 repetitions.

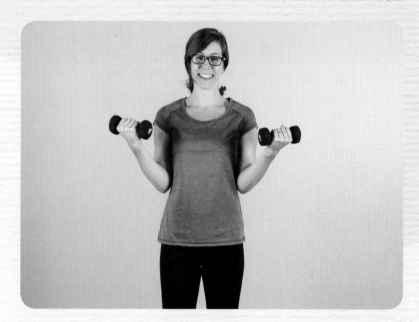

LATERAL RAISE

Lateral raises are a low-intensity, no-impact exercise. This exercise strengthens the shoulder muscles that are used for lifting and rotating the arms.

STEP 1

Stand (or sit) tall, feet at hip distance. Put arms straight down by sides, palms turned in toward body.

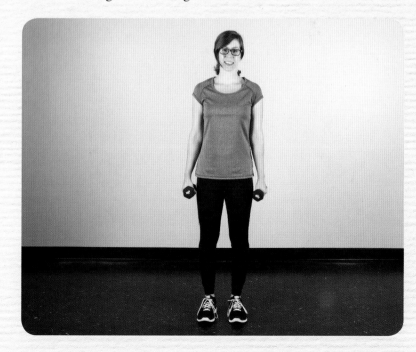

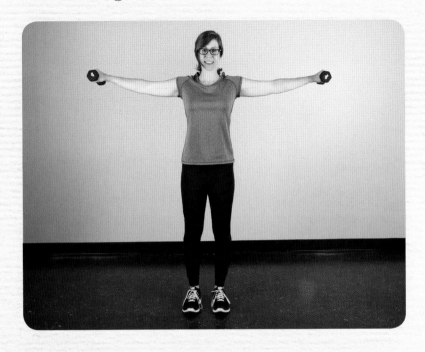

STEP 2

Lift one or both arms out to side, elbows slightly bent. Do not lift higher than the shoulder joint. Do 10–15 repetitions.

CHEST PRESS

This exercise is a low-intensity, no-impact exercise. The chest press will strengthen the chest muscles, which are important for pushing movements. This group of muscles also aids in maintaining good posture.

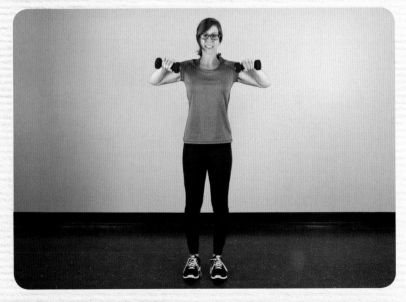

STEP 1

Stand (or sit) tall, feet at hip distance. Hands should be at chest height, palms facing down, elbows out.

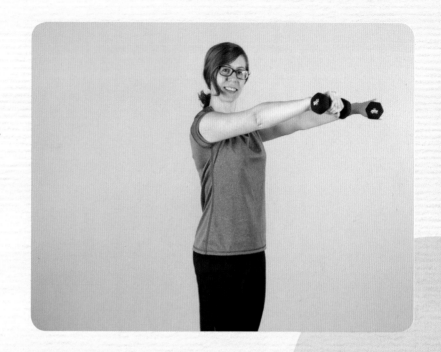

STEP 2

Press arms forward.
Do not lock elbows.

STEP 3

Return to start
position. Do
10–15 repetitions.

PRESS BACK

The press back exercise is a low-intensity, no-impact exercise. This exercise strengthens the upper back muscles, which are important for pulling movements. This group of muscles also aids in maintaining good posture.

STEP 1

Stand (or sit)
tall, feet at hip
distance. Arms
should be straight
down by sides.

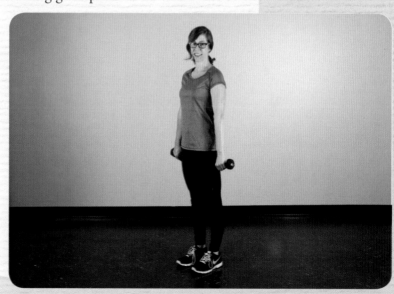

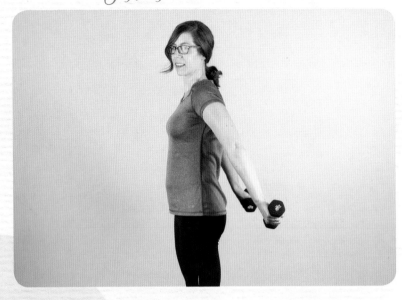

STEP 2

Face palms backward. Lift one or both arms back, squeezing shoulder blades. Keep shoulders relaxed. Do 10–15 repetitions.

SIDE LEANS

This exercise is a low-intensity, no-impact exercise. Side leans strengthen the muscles at the sides of the waist, which are part of the "core" muscle group. The core muscles aid in bending and twisting the midsection of the body. This group of muscles also contributes to posture maintenance and improving balance.

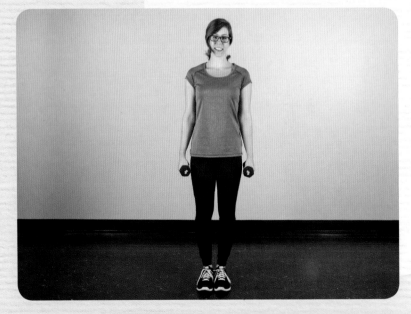

STEP 1

Stand (or sit) tall, abdominals pulled in. Arms should be straight down by sides, with the spine as straight as possible.

STEP 2

Keeping the spine long, lean to the right, crunching side of waist.

STEP 3

Do 10–15 repetitions. Repeat on other side.

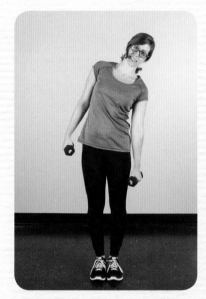
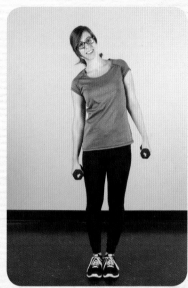

CRUNCHES

Crunches are a low-intensity, no-impact exercise. This exercise strengthens the front of the abdominals, which are part of the "core" muscle group. The front of the abdominals are the muscles responsible for bending forward; they also aid in posture maintenance and improving balance. Be cautious of this exercise if osteoporosis of the spine is present. This exercise can be done seated or laying on the floor.

IN CHAIR

STEP 1

Sit tall with abdominals pulled in.

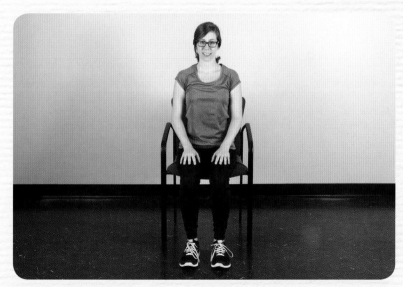

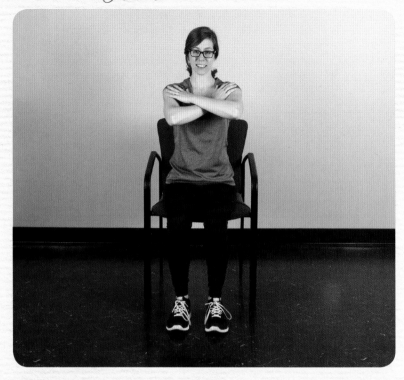

STEP 2

Cross arms in front of chest.

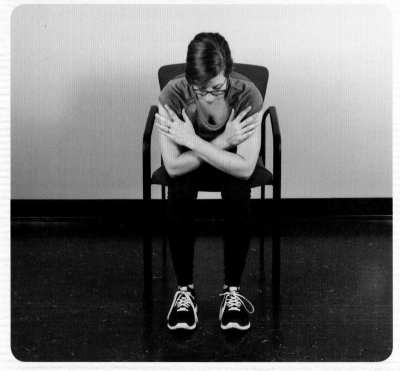

STEP 3

Keeping abdominals tight, bend forward to tap elbows to knees. Keep lower back pressing into chair. Do 10–15 repetitions.

ON THE FLOOR

STEP 1

Lie on floor, knees bent, feet flat. Place hands behind head for neck support.

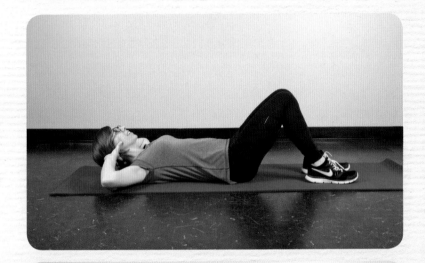

STEP 2

Keeping abdominals tight, press lower back into floor, curling head and shoulders up.

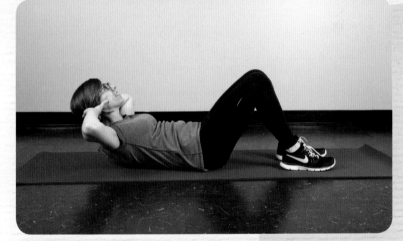

STEP 3

Do not pull on neck. Do not lift your lower back off floor.

STEP 4

Return to start position. Do 10–15 repetitions.

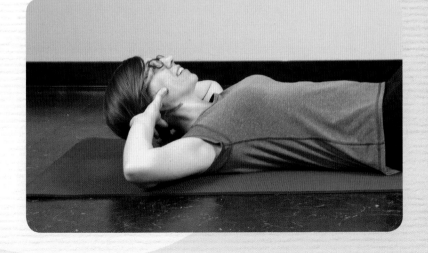

DEAD LIFT

This is a moderate-intensity, no-impact exercise. Dead lifts strengthen the muscles that run along the spine, which are important for posture maintenance and balance. Even though these muscles are located on the back, they are still an important part of the "core" muscle group. Be cautious of this exercise if lower back pain or spinal stenosis is present.

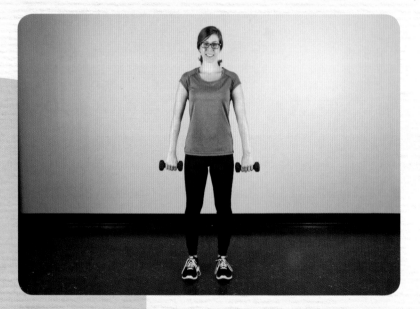

STEP 1

Stand (or sit) tall, abdominals pulled in. Arms should be hanging straight down by sides, palms facing backward.

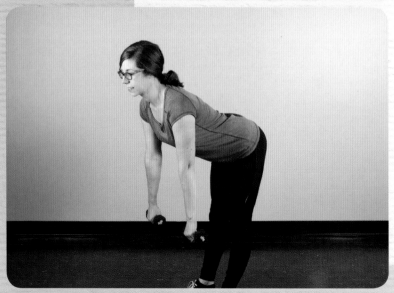

STEP 2

Keeping arms straight, bend forward with straight spine until body is at a 90 degree angle.

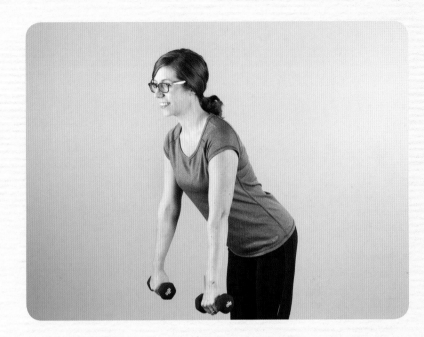

STEP 3

Press weight down through heels (hips, if seated). Slowly lift upper body back to start position. Do 10–15 repetitions.

KNEE LIFT

Knee lifts are a low-intensity, low-impact exercise. This exercise strengthens the hip muscles. Be cautious of this exercise if hip pain or injury is present. An ankle weight can be used.

STEP 1

Stand (or sit) tall. Lift bent left knee to hip height.

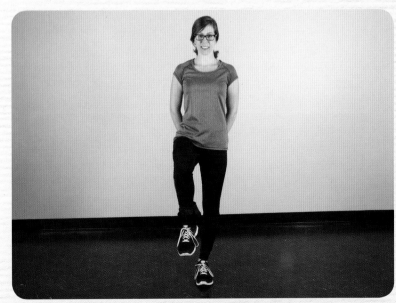

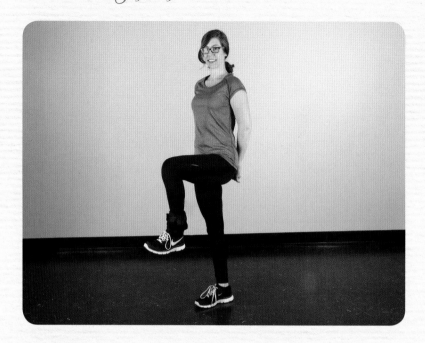

STEP 2

Keep foot flexed. Do 10–15 repetitions.

STEP 3

Repeat with other leg.

FORWARD KICK

This exercise is a low-intensity, low-impact exercise. Forward kicks strengthen the thigh muscle. Be cautious of this exercise if knee pain or injury is present. An ankle weight can be used.

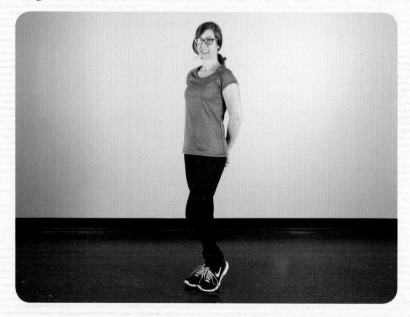

STEP 1

Stand (or sit) tall. Slightly bend knee, placing toe of left foot on floor. If seated, begin with knees bent, feet flat.

STEP 2

Straighten leg;
focus on squeezing
thigh. Do
10–15 repetitions.

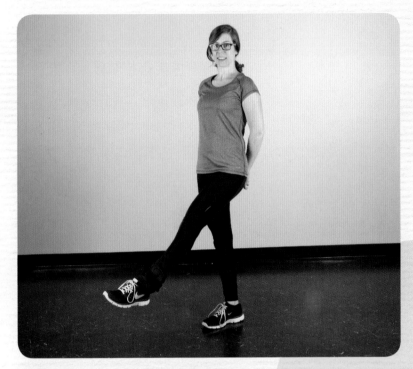

STEP 3

Repeat with
other leg.

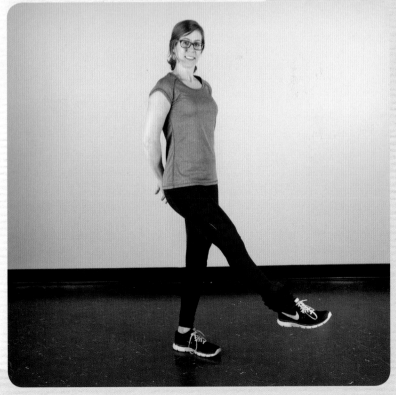

LEG CURL

The leg curl exercise is a low-intensity, no-impact exercise. This exercise strengthens the muscles at the back of the thigh, which are important for bending the knee and walking. Be cautious if knee pain or injury is present. An ankle weight can be used.

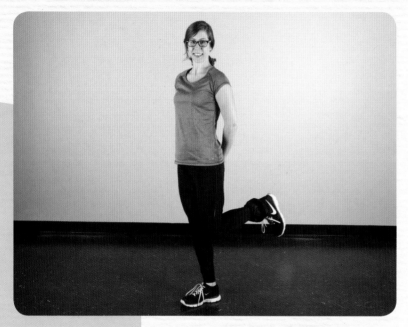

STEP 1

Stand tall, feet at hip distance. With left foot flexed, bend left knee, bringing foot backward.

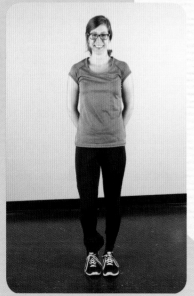
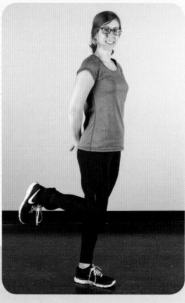

STEP 2

Keep knees close together. Lower to start position. Do 10–15 repetitions. Repeat with other leg.

SIDE LEG RAISE

This exercise is a low-intensity, no-impact exercise. Side raises strengthen the inner and outer thigh muscles, which are important for side to side movements. Be caution of this exercise if hip pain or injury is present.

STEP 1

Stand tall, feet at hip distance. Keeping upper body tall, lift straight leg to the side. Keep foot relaxed.

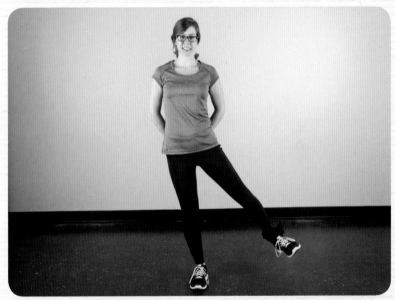

STEP 2

Return to start position. Do 10–15 repetitions.

STEP 3

Repeat with other leg.

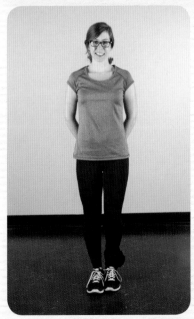
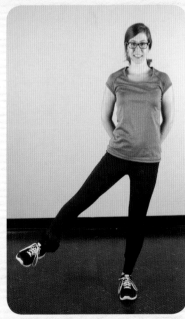

HEEL RAISES

Heel raises are a low-intensity, low-impact exercise. This exercise strengthens the calf muscles. If neuropathy of the foot is present, do this exercise seated.

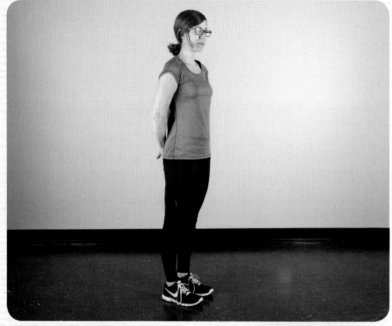

STEP 1

Stand (or sit) tall, feet at hip distance.

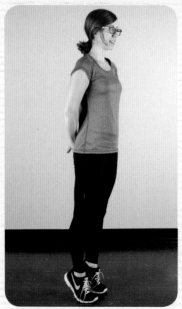
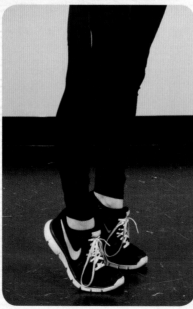

STEP 2

Keeping upper body tall and legs straight (knees bent, if seated), lift one or both heels off the ground. Do 10–15 repetitions.

SQUATS

Squats are a moderate-intensity, no-impact exercise. Squats challenge all of the muscles of the upper leg, which are important for the fundamental movements of the lower body, such as walking, bending the knees, lifting the legs, and getting in and out of a chair. If hip or knee problems are present, do partial squats or avoid this exercise.

STEP 1

Stand with feet at hip distance. Pull in abdominals to protect lower back.

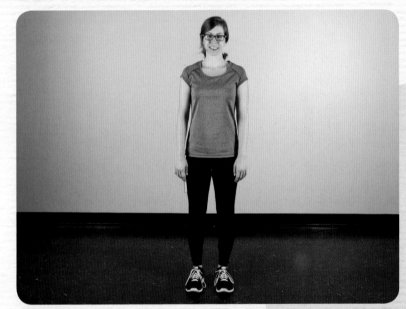

STEP 2

Bend knees and move hips back, as if sitting in a chair. Do not take knees further forward than toes.

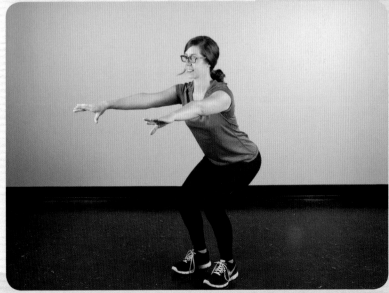

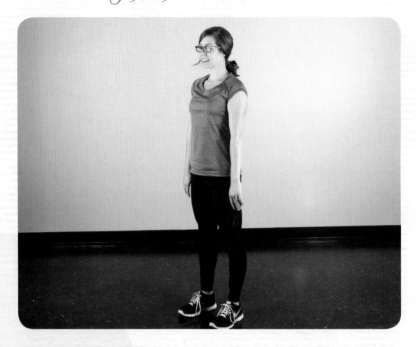

STEP 3

Press weight through heels to return to standing position. Do 10–15 repetitions.

LUNGES

Lunges are a moderate-intensity, no-impact exercise. This exercise strengthens the muscles of the thigh. If knee pain or injury is present, avoid this exercise.

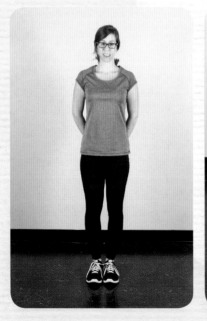

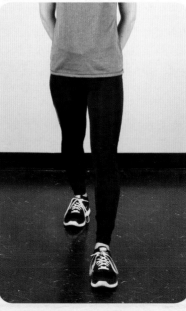

STEP 1

Stand tall with feet at hip distance. Step left foot forward into staggered stance.

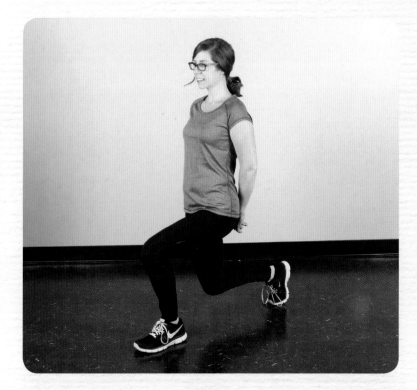

STEP 2

Keeping upper body tall, bend both knees to 90 degrees. Do not let knees go past the toes.

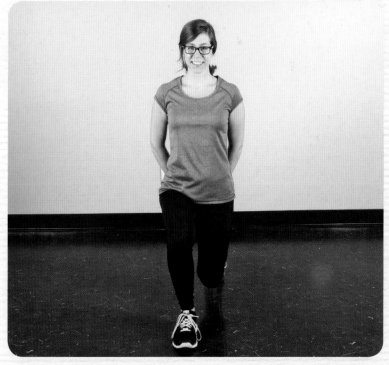

STEP 3

Return to standing position. Do 10–15 repetitions.

STEP 4

Repeat with other leg.

YOGA POSES

MOUNTAIN POSE

Mountain Pose is a low-intensity pose that is safe for all fitness levels. This exercise is beneficial for improving posture and lower body strength, as well as strengthening the core.

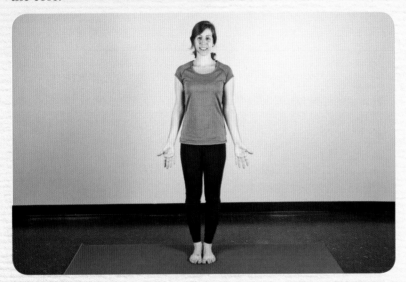

STEP 1

Stand tall with feet at hip distance. Tuck tailbone in and pull abdominals in toward spine. Relax shoulders; let arms hang by sides with palms facing out.

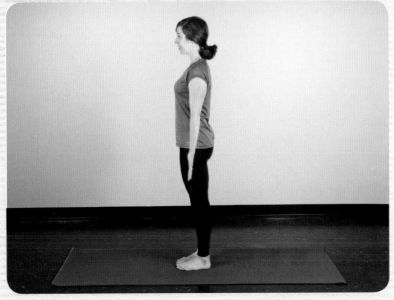

STEP 2

Reach crown of head toward the ceiling while pushing heels down into floor. Hold for 5 breaths.

LOW LUNGE/HIGH LUNGE

Low Lunge is a low-intensity balance pose. This pose may be difficult for people with peripheral neuropathy, so practice with caution. Low Lunge strengthens the lower body as well as relieving pressure caused by sciatica. High Lunge is a moderate-intensity balance pose that aids in stretching the groin and strengthens the legs.

STEP 1

Begin in Mountain Pose. Step right foot back into a wide leg stance.

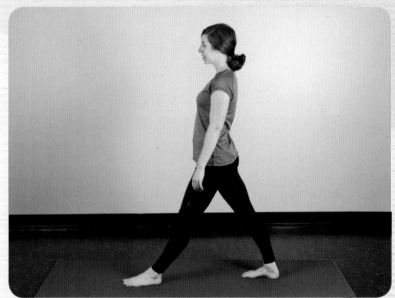

STEP 2

Bend left knee to 90 degrees while lowering left knee to floor. Straighten left leg as much as possible, pressing hips down toward floor.

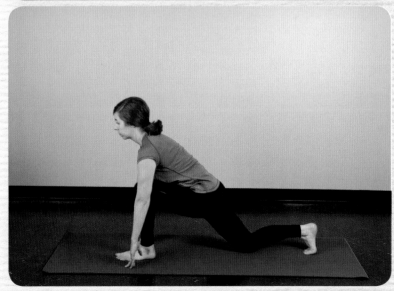

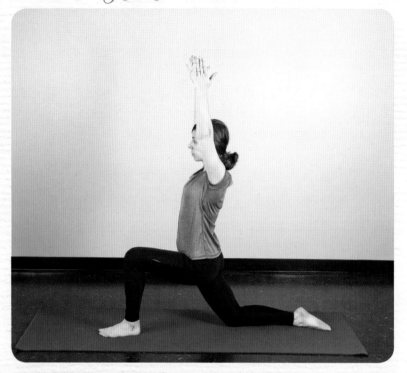

STEP 3

Place both hands on left knee and straighten upper body. Inhale while sweeping both hands up to the ceiling. For an added balance challenge, look up. Hold for 3 deep breaths. Repeat with left leg.

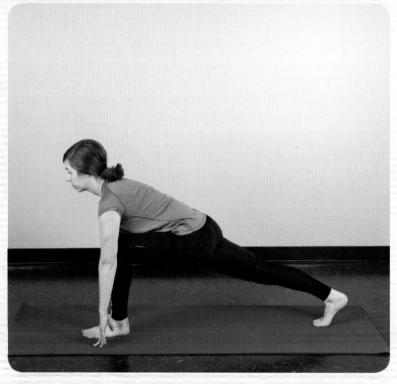

STEP 4

To move into High Lunge, place fingers on floor for stability and press right leg straight. Repeat steps 2 and 3.

DOWNWARD FACING DOG

Downward Facing Dog is a moderate-intensity pose. It strengthens and stretches muscles of the entire body and aids in preventing osteoporosis. Benefits include improved digestion and increased energy. Be cautious practicing this pose if carpal tunnel syndrome is present.

STEP 1

Begin on hands and knees with wrists under shoulders and knees under hips.

STEP 2

Curling toes under, press hips up to ceiling.

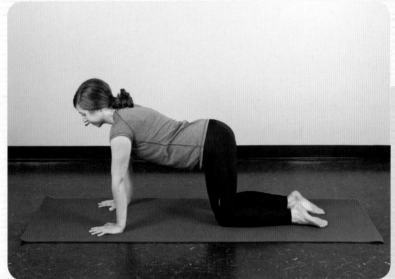

STEP 3

Adjust body so arms are straight with palms pressing firmly into floor.

STEP 4

Continue to lift hips up while pressing heels down. Bend knees slightly if pain is felt in legs. Hold for 5 breaths.

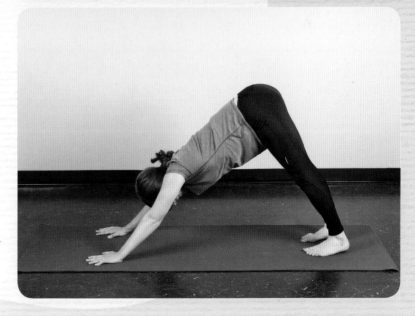

WARRIOR POSE

Warrior Pose is a moderate-intensity pose designed to strengthen and stretch the legs and ankles. This pose also facilitates core strengthening and balance training. If problems with the neck are present do not turn to look over the fingertips, but keep head forward.

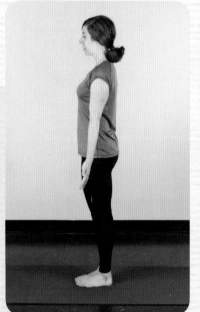
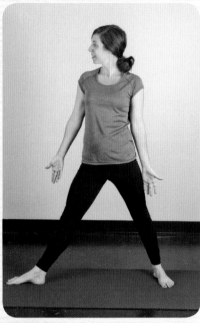

STEP 1

Begin in Mountain Pose. Step feet into wide leg stance, about 3–4 feet apart.

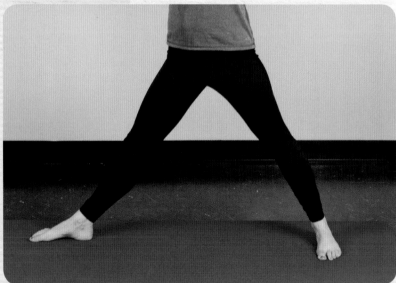

STEP 2

Turn left foot and knee outward, while right foot remains in place.

STEP 3

Inhale to sweep arms out to sides and look over fingertips.

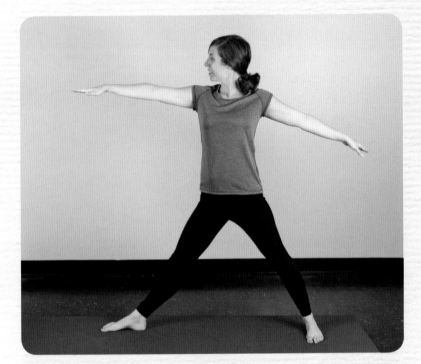

STEP 4

Bend front leg to 90 degrees. Keep upper body very tall.

STEP 5

Keeping back leg very straight, push outside edge of back foot into floor. Hold for 3 breaths.

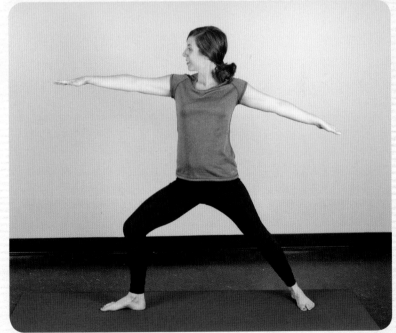

TREE POSE

This pose is a moderate-intensity balance pose. Tree Pose strengthens the ankles, calves, and thighs. It also promotes strengthening of the core and back. Tree Pose also helps improve focus.

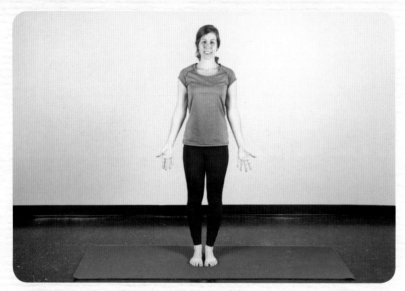

STEP 1

Begin in Mountain Pose. Rest bottom of right foot against left ankle with knee turned out. If turning knee out causes pain in hip, keep knee pointing forward.

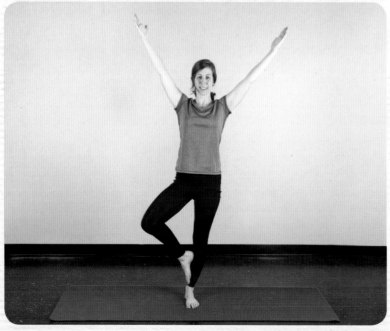

STEP 2

Keep spine long and abdominals firm. Pull right foot up to shin or thigh. Do not rest foot against knee. Reach both hands up to ceiling. Hold for 3 deep breaths. Repeat with other leg.

MOON POSE

Moon pose is a low-intensity pose used to stretch the arms and the sides of the waist.

STEP 1

Begin in Mountain Pose. Interlace fingers and turn palms down.

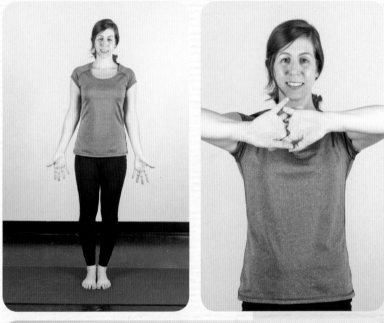

STEP 2

Inhale hands up over head, palms facing up.

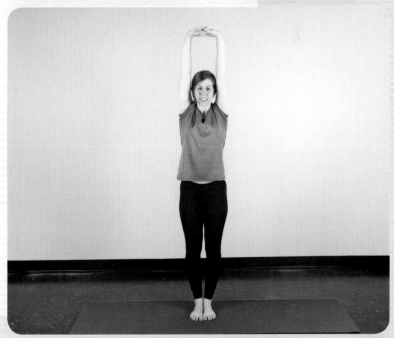

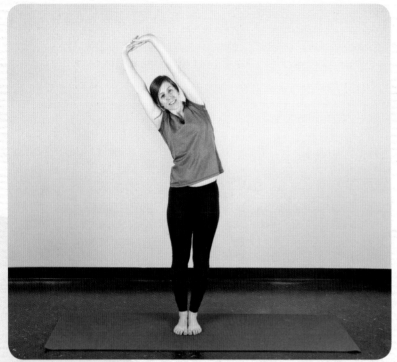

STEP 3

With hands reaching up, lean upper body to the right. Hold for 3 deep breaths.

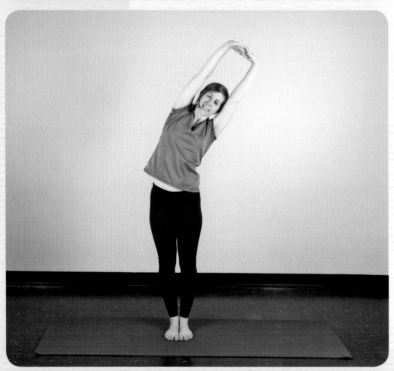

STEP 4

Repeat on left side.

CAT/COW

This flow series is low intensity and aids in strengthening and stretching the low back and core muscles. Cat and Cow is a pose used to practice pairing breath with movement, which helps relieve anxiety. Because this pose is done on hands and knees, be cautious if knee or wrist pain occurs.

ON A MAT

STEP 1

Begin on hands and knees, with wrists under shoulders and knees under hips.

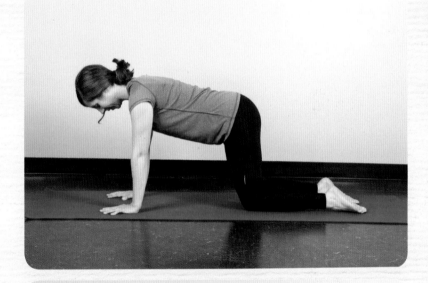

STEP 2

Inhale while rounding the back.

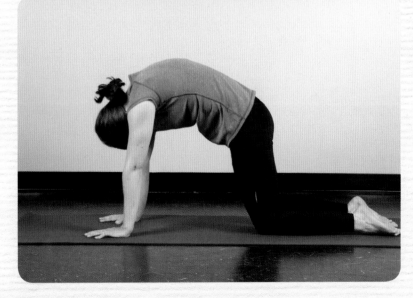

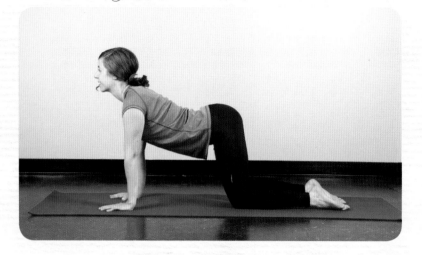

STEP 3

Exhale while pressing hands and knees into floor, arching back, and looking upward. Each breath pattern equals one set. Continue for 5 sets.

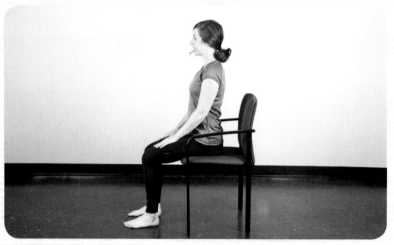

IN A CHAIR

STEP 1

Begin seated in chair with hands on thighs.

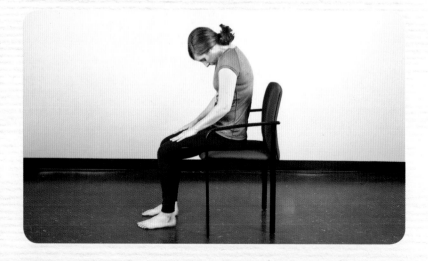

STEP 2

Inhale while rounding the back.

STEP 3

Exhale while arching back and looking up to ceiling. Each breath pattern equals one set. Continue for 5 sets.

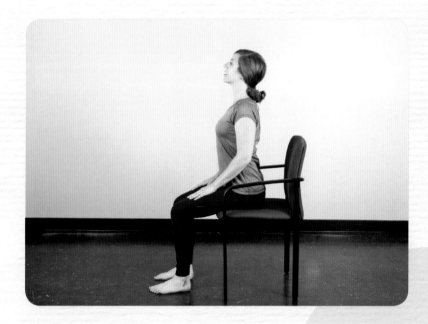

TRIANGLE POSE

Triangle Pose is a moderate-intensity pose that stretches and strengthens the lower body. It is also helpful in relieving anxiety and stress. If neck pain occurs in this stretch, do not look up at ceiling, but keep head pointing forward.

STEP 1

Begin in Mountain Pose. Step feet into wide leg stance, about 3–4 feet apart. Position feet as shown here.

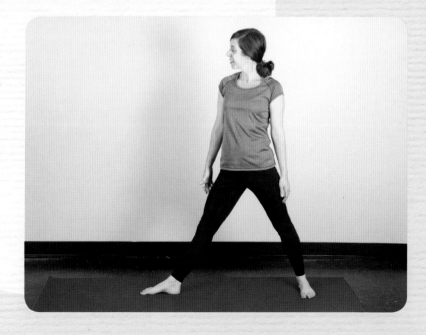

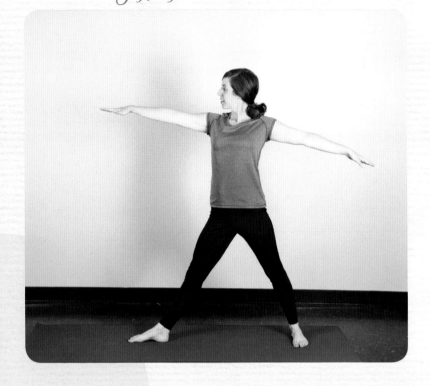

STEP 2

Inhale arms out
to sides.

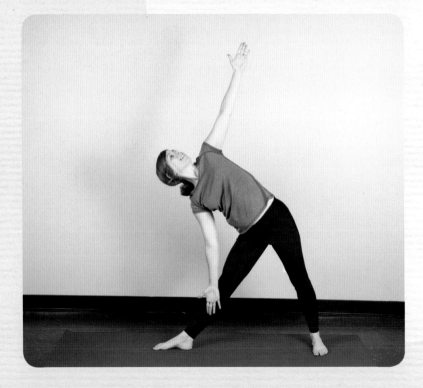

STEP 3

Exhale to reach
right hand to
shin or ankle. Left
arm reaches up to
the ceiling. If it's
comfortable, turn
the head to look
up at left arm.
Keep back
straight, tailbone
tucked under.

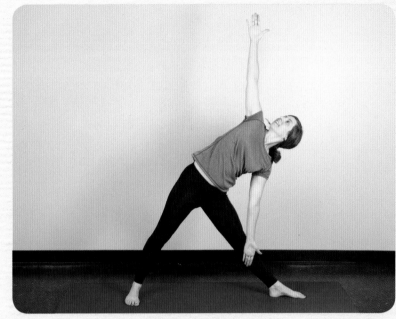

STEP 4

Hold for 3 deep breaths, then repeat on other side.

BOUND ANGEL POSE

This pose is a low-intensity pose that promotes stimulation of the heart and improves circulation. Other benefits include decreased stress, anxiety, and depression. Bound Angel Pose focuses on stretching the inner thigh, groin, and knees. If hip, groin, or knee pain is present, sit up on a pillow or yoga block.

STEP 1

Sit tall with feet flat on floor, knees bent.

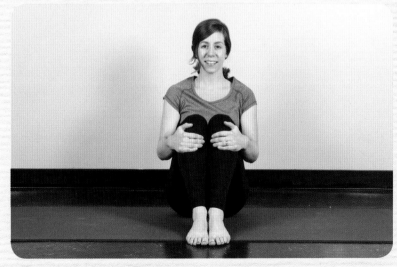

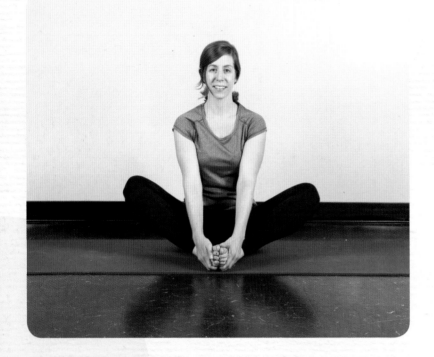

STEP 2

Open knees out to sides and pull heels in toward pelvis.

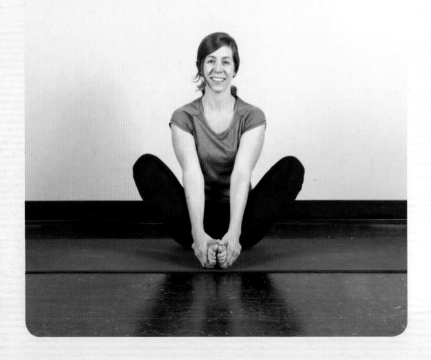

STEP 3

Place hands around feet.

STEP 4

Round forward, bringing head towards feet. Hold for 3 deep breaths.